FINGEROLOGY

THE COMPLETE GUIDE TO THE FINGERS

HILLARY J. KENER
AND
MICHAEL ZEIDE M.D.

WITH ELANA ZEIDE

iUNIVERSE, INC.
BLOOMINGTON

FINGEROLOGY
The Complete Guide to the Fingers

The information, ideas, and suggestions in this book are not intended as a substitute for professional medical advice. Before following any suggestions contained in this book, you should consult your personal physician. Neither the author nor the publisher shall be liable or responsible for any loss or damage allegedly arising as a consequence of your use or application of any information or suggestions in this book.

iUniverse books may be ordered through booksellers or by contacting:

iUniverse
1663 Liberty Drive
Bloomington, IN 47403
www.iuniverse.com
1-800-Authors (1-800-288-4677)

Because of the dynamic nature of the Internet, any Web addresses or links contained in this book may have changed since publication and may no longer be valid. The views expressed in this work are solely those of the author and do not necessarily reflect the views of the publisher, and the publisher hereby disclaims any responsibility for them.

ISBN: 978-1-4401-6703-4 (sc)
ISBN: 978-1-4401-6705-8 (dj)
ISBN: 978-1-4401-6704-1 (ebk)

Library of Congress Control Number: 2010912779

Printed in the United States of America

iUniverse rev. date: 11/16/2010

Rose is a rose is a rose is a rose
Loveliness extreme.
Extra gaiters,
Loveliness extreme.
Sweetest ice-cream,
Pages ages page ages page ages

- Gertrude Stein, *Sacred Emily (1913)*

A rose by any other name would smell as sweet.

-Shakespeare

PREFACE

According to the Global Population Profile, by 2012, there will be 71 billion fingers in the world.

The Question: What are the names of the fingers?

    A. The fingers should be named: thumb, index finger, middle finger, ring finger, and little finger.

    B. The naming of the fingers is iconic- and often, idiosyncratic and paradoxical.

    C. The naming of the fingers varies from childhood nursery rhymes to individual cultural backgrounds, life- experiences, between different musical instruments, and other activities.

    D. All of the above

The Answer: **D. All of the above**

Nomenclature – the names or terms comprising a set or system – is part of the universal language of a society. However, language is often an imperfect form of communication. It is recognized that words can change in denotation and connotation by contextual modifiers, i.e., the meaning of a word can be different in different situations.

Consequently, this may create serious problems in communications and consensus among different groups with varied backgrounds and perceptions. The meaning of a word can be distorted by personal experiences and context. Individuals may interpret the language differently, leading to confusion and errors in communication when the basic concept or subject is in fact the same.

INTRODUCTION

Intuitively and inherently we all perceive "we know" the names of our fingers. But finger naming is not intuitive.

The instinctive simplicity of this subject – **naming the fingers** – is actually confusing and complex.

In T.S. Eliot's classic, *The Naming of Cats*, (from "Old Possum's Book of Practical Cats"):

> ***The naming of cats is a difficult matter,***
> *It isn't just one of your holiday games;*
> *You may think at first I'm mad as a hatter*
> *When I tell you a cat must have three*
> *different names.*

Paraphrasing T.S. Eliot, **the naming of fingers is a difficult matter.**

What are the names of the finger? **The fingers should be named: thumb, index finger, middle finger, ring finger, and little finger.**

But this is answer is not always correct, complete, or adequate; at times, there is a confusion and aberrations.

Ironically, the naming of the fingers is iconic- and often, idiosyncratic and paradoxical. The naming of the fingers varies from childhood nursery rhymes to individual cultural backgrounds, life-experiences, between different musical instruments, and other activities.

The most significant mistake is to make a distinction for the thumb from the other fingers. Thus, the index finger is erroneously referred to as the 1ˢᵗ finger, and the middle finger as the 2ⁿᵈ finger, etc.

Unfortunately, these misconceptions are still pervasive and perpetuated by the media. For example, from the Simple English Wikipedia web site, the definition of "thumb," references "the thumb and the 4 fingers."

A Google search for the definition of the "middle finger," leads to the link:

> <u>The Free Dictionary by Farlex:</u>
> **Noun 1. middle finger** - *the second finger; between the index finger and the ring finger*
> *finger - any of the terminal members of the hand (sometimes excepting the thumb); "her fingers were long and thin"*

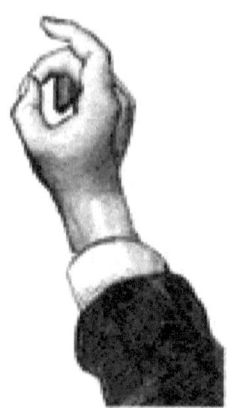

As illustrated above, the middle finger is incorrectly defined as "the second finger, between the index and the ring finger."

Paradoxically, the index is the **2ⁿᵈ finger for a pianist; yet, guitarists refer to the index finger as the 1ˢᵗ finger.**

Rhetorically, we reiterate that the fingers should be called by their proper name and not numerically.

Nonetheless, to the FBI, when fingerprinting, **the right index finger is Finger #2 and the left index finger is Finger #7.**

Making string figures is an art involving the intricate looping, bending, and extension of strings of various lengths. In this game, **the left index finger is designated as L-2.**

Yet in the rhyme and rote of the nursery rhyme, "Tommie Thumb" children are taught that **the index finger is "Mr. Pointer Man"; however, in Palmistry, the index finger is the "Jupiter finger."**

Symbolically, the index finger can be a directional signal, or inspirational as in Michelangelo's masterpiece, "Sistine Chapel," or raised as a victory gesture – and simply, holding the index finger up and stationary means, "wait." The same index finger when brought close to the lips conveys, "Be quiet!"

But with the hand held palm out and the thumb and middle fingers touching, it represents the **letter *d*** in the American Sign Language alphabet.

Moreover and most importantly, in medicine there have been serious consequences from a lack of uniform specificity in naming the fingers, resulting in wrote site and wrong-sided surgery.

Medical students are instructed that anatomically the index finger should be called the "index finger." Yet, when surgeons are coding surgical procedures for submission for payment, the regulatory requirement mandates that the **right index finger must be coded as F6 and the left index finger as F1.**

Anecdotally, a colleague, an internationally renowned Hand Surgeon, raised in Iran, recalls that as a young foreign medical doctor he had an unusual encounter in the emergency room at George Washington Hospital, in Washington, DC. Dr. "M.M." was a new intern called in to evaluate a patient who had sustained a severe traumatic injury to her left 5th toe. He explained to the patient that they would have to perform surgery on the "5th finger"- not realizing that the translation of Farsi for toe, equivalent in English, was "finger of the foot." She was irate, agitated and requested a more senior doctor.

Currently, many doctors and other Health Care Providers still inadvertently in their reports (e.g., radiology) or colloquially refer to the fingers as the 1st digit or 1st finger; or 2nd digit; or 3rd digit; or 4th digit, and the thumb as the thumb. Whereas others refer to the thumb as the 1st digit or 1st ray or 1st finger, and the index finger as the 2nd digit, etc.

In other words, some health care providers still inaccurately consider the thumb as separate and distinct – not a finger- and in contradistinction to the numerical order of the fingers, without realizing the potential consequences.

Retrospectively, in 1969, in the second issue of a new British journal, The Hand, Dr. H. Graham Stack, wrote a classic article, "Naming the Fingers," elaborating on these confusions, ambiguities, and misconceptions.

With the permission of the Sage Publications, we have reproduced the article- and it is just as relevant today as it was four decades ago. The lessons that were illustrated and preached have still been relatively ignored. Indeed, it may be more relevant as the problem of "Naming the Fingers" has not been resolved or eliminated- and there have been over 200 reports of wrong site surgery on the hand in 2007 in the US. – including 123 on the fingers.

While various organizations and institutions, including the American Academy of Orthopaedic Surgeons, the American Association for Surgery of the Hand, and the Joint Commission (an independent organization that accredits and certifies health care organizations), have made various proposals and protocols to address this situation, but the problem still persists and places a black mark on the medical profession.

This book has evolved into a reference book, a compendium for "fingers."

On a lighter side, we decided to have some fun and compiled and incorporated a collection of diverse and interesting facts, concepts, symbols, and clichés about the fingers; including anatomy, the nomenclature for finger strings, idioms, slang, and general trivia.

We hope the reader finds the materials curious, interesting, educational, and enjoyable.

*If any term, word, cliché, or phrase is not in this book, we would like to know so we can include it in the next edition.

Please add any additions, corrections, or suggestions at <u>Fingerology. com</u>.

ACKNOWLEDGMENTS

We would like to recognize and show our appreciation to the following:

- **American Society for Surgery of the Hand (ASSH)** for use of their graphics. The mission of the American Society for Surgery of the Hand (ASSH) is to advance the science and practice of hand surgery through education, research and advocacy on behalf of patients and practitioners. Founded in 1946, the American Society for Surgery of the Hand is the oldest medical specialty society in the United States devoted entirely to continuing medical education related to hand surgery.

- **Andrew Kener** for his editorial assistance and intellectual analysis.

- **Anne Massey** who designed the Palmistry picture of the hand and fingers. It is a terrific picture! Her web site is www. astrologicallyspeaking.com

- **Bartleby.com** for kindly allowing us to reproduce the 1918 edition of "Gray's Anatomy" section on the hand and fingers. It is hard to reinvent the wheel- and Gray's Anatomy is the gold standard. Since its incorporation in 1999 and the release of preeminent contemporary reference works, Bartleby.com has become the most comprehensive reference publisher on the web, meeting the needs of students, educators, and the intellectually curious.

- **Changingminds.org** for use of their article on "finger body language".

- **Consulates and embassies** of all of the countries who contributed to the language section of our book.

- **Donna Zeide M.D.,** a dermatologist, for her contribution to the fingernail segment.

- **Joseph Chalal M.D.,** a friend and colleague who provided the support and encouragement to reach for excellence. – and encouragement for this and other projects.

- **László A. Magyar**, author of DIGITUS MEDICINALIS – THE ETYMOLOGY OF THE NAME, a very well researched article about naming of the ring finger. It was brilliantly written and researched.

- **Leslie Zemenek** for her vast knowledge about Palmistry. She is an inspiration for her profession and professionalism.

- **Mas Masoumi M.D.,** a very skilled hand surgeon, a doctor's doctor.

- **Primal Pictures** has a series of 3D Anatomy graphics that feature highly detailed, interactive 3D computer graphic models of various anatomical structures. We thank them for their exceptional anatomy pictures that they allowed us to reproduce. A century ago, Henry Gray's anatomical illustrations were the standard. Today, Primal Pictures has set the new standard.

- **SAGE Publications** is an independent international publisher of journals and books. Known for their commitment to quality and innovation, SAGE's prestigious and highly cited journals are available electronically on the award winning *SAGE Journals Online*

- **Taylor Pong and Alex Maniotis and Christopher Castillo** and the other teenage kids that helped with the filing, sorting, organization, and typing, etc. They were enthusiastic, energetic, and supportive.

- **WikiHow** is "a collaborative writing project to build the world's largest, highest quality how-to manual."

- **Wikipedia** is a "free multilingual, open content encyclopedia project operated by the non-profit Wikimedia Foundation. Its name is a portmanteau of the words *wiki* (a technology for creating collaborative websites) and *encyclopedia*. Launched in 2001 by Jimmy Wales and Larry Sanger, it attempts to collect and summarize all human knowledge in every major language." Wikipedia is the largest individual active reference site on the internet. We utilized some terms and concepts from this site; however there are errors in Wikipedia that we have pointed out - and will edit on Wikipedia's web site in the future.

DEDICATIONS

In memory of H. Graham Stack, an extraordinary English physician and pioneer in hand surgery. The authors express our sincere appreciation and gratitude for his professional passion and enormous contributions to Hand Surgery. His article in 1969, _Naming the Fingers_, inspired our efforts in this book.

Peter Mark Roget, a British physician and lexicographer. In 1852, he published the _Thesaurus of English Words and Phrases_. Our book is a "thesaurus" about fingers.

To my parents, Donna and Morris Kener, whom I love and admire, and to my amazing brother Andrew.

To Denise, my wife: brilliant, beautiful, special and extraordinary.

To our parents and family who inspire us to pursue excellence-and especially to Dr. Harold and Stella Zeide. Grandpa Harold is the inspiration and Grandma Stella is the heart and soul of a wonderful family.

Elana Zeide, a brilliant and beautiful renaissance person, and the creative inspiration for this project.

-Hillary Kener

-Michael Zeide

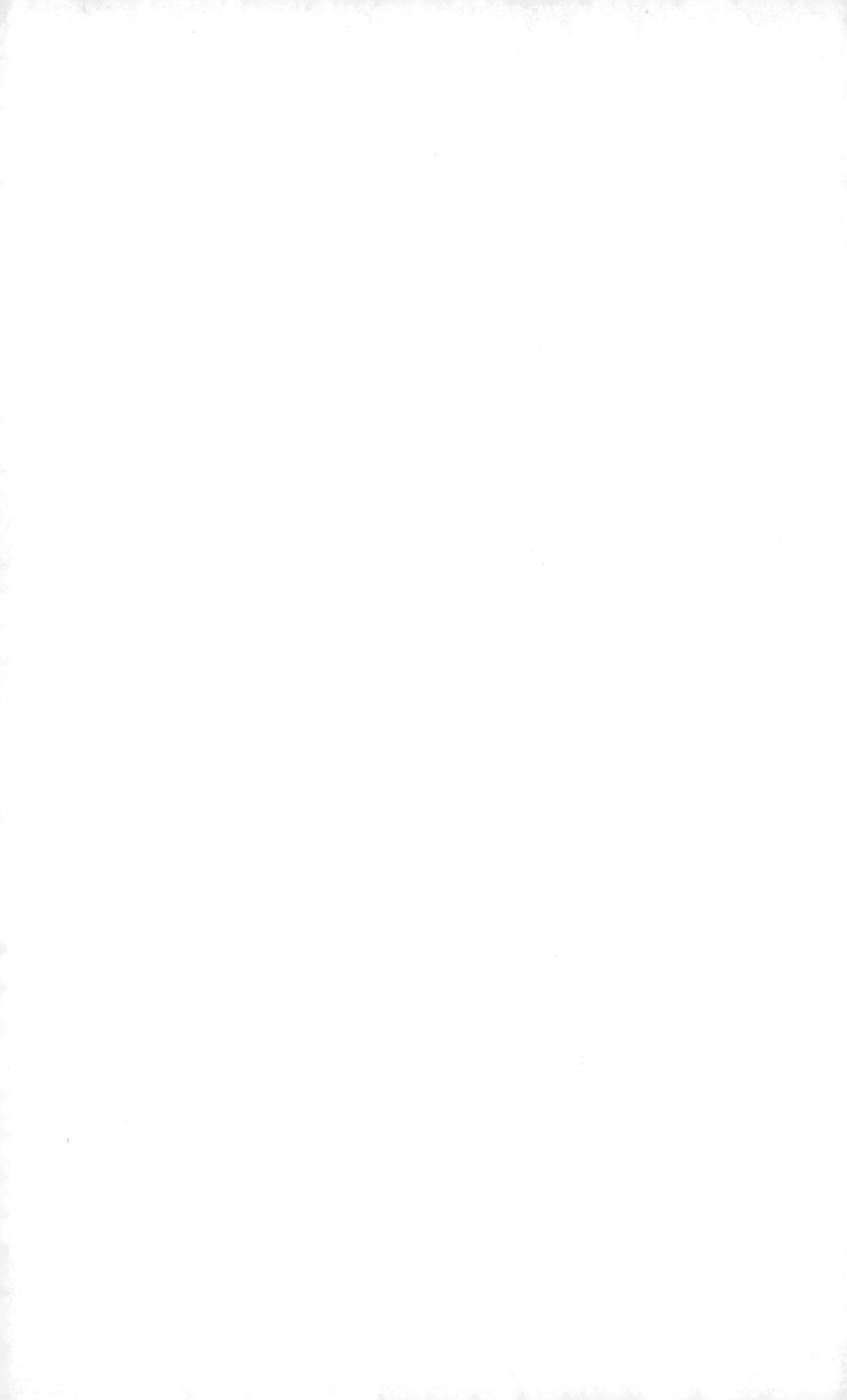

NAMING THE FINGERS
H. GRAHAM STACK, LONDON

Repetition of the need to use the standard names for the fingers is necessary to reduce the continued mistakes in Surgery due to confusion of nomenclature.

DEFINITIONS

Oxford English Dictionary

The Shorter Oxford English Dictionary (1933) under the heading The Finger, gives the following:-

Finger. Com. Teut: Old English finger: Old Teutonic fingro-z perh: comm: W pre-Teut penge Five.

One of the five terminal members of the hand: especially one of the four excluding the thumb.

The fingers are five in number, in each hand. They are named thumb, index, middle, ring and little fingers. 1861, forefinger: the index finger.

Nomina Anatomica

The Nomina Anatomica (1966), the third edition of the Paris Nomina Anatomica (P.N.A.) abbreviated to the N.A., gives the following (p. 19):-

Digiti Manus

Pollex   (Digitus I)
Index   (Digitus II)

Digitus Medius (Digitus III)
Digitus anularis* (Digitus IV)
Digitus minimus (Digitus V)

The names approved by the anatomists are clearly those translated as index, middle, ring, and little. The numbering is clear and logical•

It would be dangerous therefore to refer to Digitus II as the first finger.

* Note.-N.A.p. 12 note 3: Anulus. It was agreed that this term should be spelt with one "n" and not two, as the latter is apparently incorrect.

PROFESSIONAL ADVICE

The Secretary of the Medical Defence Union wrote in 1955: -

.. "To do as many do--namely to number the fingers 1, 2, 3, etc. and to record in the clinical notes, for example, that finger number 3 requires amputation --is to set the stage for a serious surgical mishap. Now and again the surgeon, reading the notes of the case at a later date, before proceeding to operate has counted wrongly by choosing to regard the thumb as number 1 instead of the index finger. In this way the wrong finger has been amputated or chosen for some other operation.

"It seems to the Council of the Union that this serious mistake would be obviated if hospital medical officers when writing up clinical notes described the actual finger affected by adopting the designations of "the thumb", "the index finger", "the middle finger", "the ring finger", and "the little finger".

In September 1960 the Secretary of the Union again wrote reiterating this point in the same terms, as in the previous twelve months the Union had dealt with nine claims where an operation had been performed on the wrong limb or digit.

In 1961 (and revised in 1966), a Joint Memorandum on Safeguards against wrong operations was produced by the Medical Defence Union, and the Royal College of Nursing, and the National Council of Nurses of the United Kingdom in which the following was written (page 6):

Suggested safeguards

I.   In order to avoid the possibility of any ambiguity concerning the finger(s) on which the operation is to be performed, the fingers should always be described as thumb, index, middle, ring and little fingers, and not as 1st, 2nd, 3rd, 4th and 5th.

This document was produced after consultation with the Minister of Health, and has the support of the Secretary of State who has regularly recommended the Memorandum to the Medical Profession for their guidance.

HISTORICAL REFERENCES

Wood-Jones (1949) quotes Diemerbroeck (1672) from his Anatome Corporis Humani: -

"The first which is the thickest, and equals all the rest for strength, is called pollex or the thumb. The second is the forefinger from the use, called the index or demonstrator, the pointer, because it is used in the demonstration of things. The third or middle finger is called impudicus, famosus, and obscoenus, the obscene and infamous, because it is usually held forth at men pointed at for infamy and in derision. The fourth, the ring finger, or annularis and medicus, the physicians finger, because that persons formerly admitted doctors of physic were wont to wear a gold ring upon that finger. The fifth called the little finger, in Latin auricularis, or earfinger, for that men generally pick their ears with it."

Bertelsen and Capener (1960) have also quoted this section and others, and made the following table of some of the more ancient names in the early Anglo- Saxon, in use in King Alfred's day.

NAMES OF THE FINGERS

	Modern English	*Alfred's Anglo-Saxon*
THUMB	Pollex	DUMA
INDEX	Forefinger, Salutatorius, Demonstratorius, Shooting, Sagittatur	SYTHE FINGER
MIDDLE	Medius, Famosus, Impudicus, Obscoenus	MIDLESTAFINGER
RING	Annulus, Medicus	GOLDFINGER
LITTLE	Minimus, Auricularis	LYTLAFINGER

THE BOOK OF THE HAND (1965)

This book by Gettings is a review of the history of Hand Reading, an illustrated history of Palmistry. From a very early period, at least the fifteenth century, the fingers have been named:-

Index The finger of Jupiter,
Middle The finger of Saturn,
Ring The finger of Apollo,
Little The finger of Mercury

OTHER LANGUAGES

In the Latin languages the names are derived from the Latin digitus, Doigt in French and Dedo in Spanish and Portuguese.

Pouce and Pulgar from Pollex.

The names are translated as follows: -

Latin	French	Spanish	Portuguese
Pollex	Pouce	Pulgar	Polegar
Index	Index	Indice	Indicador
Medius	Medius	Medio	Medio
Anularis	Annulaire	Anular	Anular
Minimus		Menique	Minimo
Auricularis	Auriculaire		

The German names are similar to the English or Anglo-Saxon, since the Teutonic Language is the basis here.

English	German
Thumb	Daumen
Index	Zeigefinger (Zeigen = show, demonstrate)
Middle	Mittelfinger
Ring	Ringfinger
Little	Kleinfinger

The Japanese consider the thumb to be one of the fingers, and call the finger by name (Tajima (1967)): oya-yubi (parent finger), hitosashi-yubi (index finger), naka-yubi (middle finger), kusuri-yubi (remedy finger) and ko-yubi (little finger).

4

The word yubi meaning a finger is considered to have been derived from an old Japanese word. Old Japanese is thought to have been derived from the Ural- Altaic language group, which is the same as Mongolian.

In medical descriptions the Japanese use dai-ichi-shi (1st digit), dai-ni-shi (2nd digit), dai-san-shi (3rd digit) etc.

The word shi is derived from old Chinese meaning digit. Thus in Japanese there are two different words, synonyms, with the same meaning, one from old Japanese, the other from old Chinese.

DIFFICULTIES

Use of Numbers

Several difficulties are inherent in the use of numbers for finger. Firstly, there are two distinct methods, represented by the difference between the piano player counting one to five, and the violinist who counts only four fingers, since the thumb is behind the instrument, and not used for the fingering.

Many people, discount the thumb as a finger, starting with the index finger as the first. Logically this would mean that the little finger should be the fourth, whereas it is almost universally called the fifth.

It is also illogical that the "first finger" (the index finger) is placed on the second metacarpal.

The only rational use of numbers is therefore to refer to the digits and rays by numbers. However there remains in this system the continued possibility that the second digit will later be referred to as the second finger, and the confusion will be continued.

It is therefore essential that in clinical surgery, the numbers should not be used except for the metacarpals, and even there, confusion will be minimised by calling the second metacarpal, the index metacarpal.

Purism

The main objection to the classical name of "middle finger" has been the pedantic difficulty of deciding which is the middle finger among four. Since there are five fingers, this difficulty should resolve itself, as it is not etymologically valid.

Dictation

There is however a source of difficulty in dictating when "middle" and "little" (or perhaps "liddle") can be misheard by a stenographer. There is a similar likelihood of confusion between "long" and "ring" in shorthand. Forefinger can be confused with "fourth finger".

Relative length

Kaplan (1966) has illustrated a hand in which the middle finger is shorter than its neighbours, and writes: "The middle finger or medius known as such for many years, was recently renamed for no apparent reason, the long finger. It may be better to retain the old established name of middle finger to avoid confusion in cases of congenital or pathologic shortening of the middle finger as shown . . . .

The Lancet (1965) summed the problem up as follows:-

.. the digits can be named after the popular fashion--thumb, index, middle, ring and little. This system may seem foolproof, but it would still behove any doctor corresponding with a colleague in remote parts to make sure that matrimony there is indeed signified by the wearing of a ring, and that this is placed on the finger next the smallest one. Some problems will defeat every scheme; and the mind recoils from those which could attend the writing of an intelligible report about a man who has lost one digit from a hand showing a six-fingered polydactyly but having no properly differentiated thumb.

SUMMARY

In order to avoid confusion, it is important that the fingers are named, rather than numbered, in Great Britain, this move has been supported by the Ministry of Health and the Medical Defence Societies, and the Royal College of Nursing, and National Council of Nurses of the United Kingdom, who all recommend the terms: Thumb, Index, Middle, Ring and Little.

Languages derived from Latin use derivatives of the Latin digitus, French doigt, and Portuguese and Spanish dedo.

German uses the term "Mittel finger" for the middle finger, and the Japanese also use "middle finger", "naka-yubi".

The English word "finger" is considered to have been derived from the pre-Teutonic word "penge" meaning five, and this means that there is no logical objection to calling the middle digit the middle finger.

As regards the sound of the names, it is possible for a stenographer to mishear "middle" as "little" or vice versa, but it is equally possible for her to confuse the shorthand versions of "ring" and "long".

It is however now clear that the great majority of languages, and of surgeons are now accepting the recommended terminology used here in this volume.

APPENDIX
LIST OF THE CAUSES OF THE FIVE OPERATIONS ON THE WRONG FINGER IN BRITAIN BETWEEN JANUARY, 1966 AND JUNE, 1969

As reported to the Medical Defence Union, and reproduced with their permission.

1. The right ring finger operated on instead of the left ring finger for a thickening of the flexor sheath. No explanation other than a mistake.

2. The nail fold of the left middle finger operated on for a septic condition instead of the right little finger. Surgeon operated on the left hand because it was presented to him. The records were correct.

3. The tendon sheath of the left flexor pollicis longus operated on instead of the right. Patient referred to Out Patients for attention to the right thumb, put down on the waiting list as a trigger left thumb, operation carried out without first checking with the patient. Consent form not completed, as to the nature of the operation.

4. Incision made over the proximal interphalangeal joint of the left middle finger instead of the left ring finger. The intention was to amputate the terminal and middle phalanges of the left ring finger due to a previous injury. The mistake was discovered only after the incision and after the digital nerve of the left middle finger had been severed on its radial side.

5. Exploration of pulp of right ring finger instead of right middle finger to remove splinter of glass. Notes and consent form incorrectly completed. X-ray not checked carefully.

REFERENCES

ADDISON, P. H. (1960) Operating on the wrong limb or digit. British Medical Journal. Vol. 2, 806.

BERTELSEN, A., and CAPENER, N. (1960) Fingers, Compensation and King Canute. Journal of Bone and Joint Surgery, 42B : 390.

DIEMERBROECK, I. DE (1672) Anatome Corporis Humani, Utrecht 754. The English translation of this work was published by William Salmon, London, 1694.

FORBES, R. (1955) Numbering of fingers. British Medical Journal, Vol. 2, 851.

GETTINGS, F. (1965) The Book of the Hand. London, Paul Hamlyn, Ltd.

JOINT MEMORANDUM on Safeguards against wrong operations (1966) Medical Defence Union, London.

KAPLAN, E. B. (1965) Functional and Surgical Anatomy of the Hand. 2nd Ed. 23. Philadelphia. J. B. Lippincott Company.

LANCET (1965) Annotation "Name this finger". Lancet, Vol. 2, 1060.

NOMINA ANATOMICA (1966) Excerpta Medica Foundation, Amsterdam.

SHORTER OXFORD ENGLISH DICTIONARY (1933) 701. Oxford, Clarendon Press.

TAJIMA, T. (1967) Personal Communication.

WOOD JONES, F. (1949) The principles of anatomy as seen in the hand. Second Edition. London, Bailliere, Tindall and Cox.

ANATOMY

The anatomy of the hand is complex, intricate, and fascinating.

The hand and fingers are composed of many different bones, muscles, joints, and ligaments that allow for a variety of movements and functions.

PALMAR SURFACE[1]

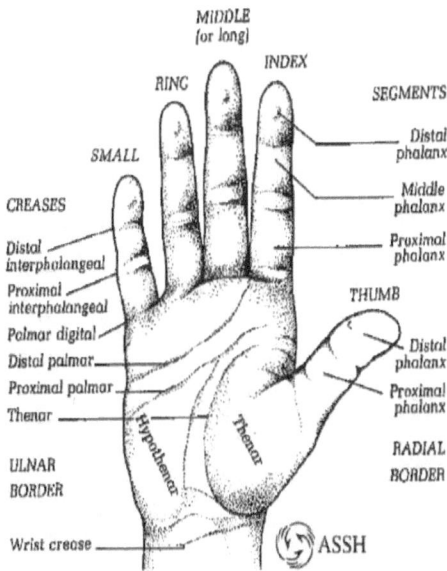

1 Images © 2002 American Society for Surgery of the Hand *Essentials of Hand Surgery*

BONES & JOINTS[2]

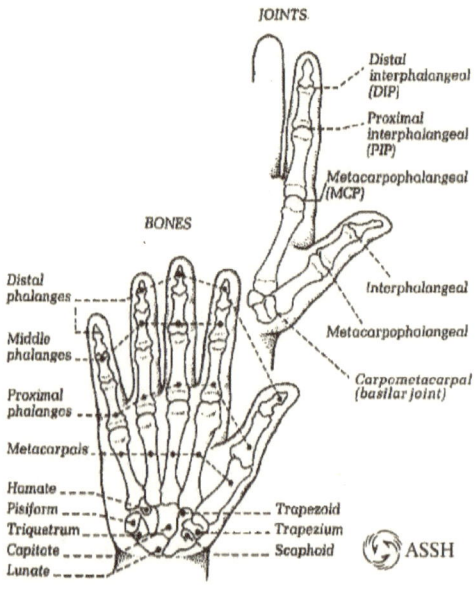

JOINTS

Distal
interphalangeal
(DIP)

Proximal
interphalangeal
(PIP)

Metacarpophalangeal
(MCP)

BONES

Interphalangeal

Metacarpophalangeal

Distal
phalanges

Carpometacarpal
(basilar joint)

Middle
phalanges

Proximal
phalanges

Metacarpals

Hamate
Pisiform
Triquetrum
Capitate
Lunate

Trapezoid
Trapezium
Scaphoid

ASSH

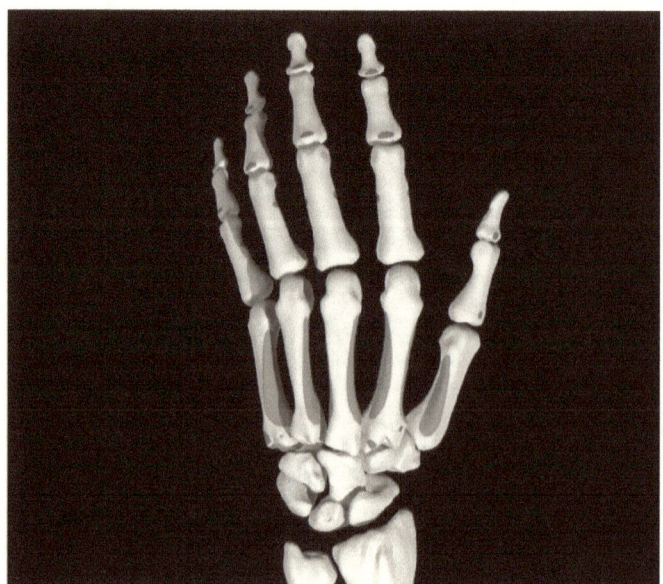

©2006 Primal Pictures

2   Images © 2002 American Society for Surgery of the Hand *Essentials of Hand Surgery*

HENRY GRAY- ANATOMY OF THE HUMAN BODY. 1918.[3]

6B. 2. THE METACARPUS

The **metacarpus** consists of five cylindrical bones which are numbered from the lateral side (*ossa metacarpalia I-V*); each consists of a body and two extremities.

Common Characteristics of the Metacarpal Bones.—The Body (*corpus; shaft*).—The body is prismoid in form, and curved, so as to be convex in the longitudinal direction behind, concave in front. It presents three surfaces: medial, lateral, and dorsal. The **medial** and **lateral surfaces** are concave, for the attachment of the Interossei, and separated from one another by a prominent anterior ridge. The **dorsal surface** presents in its distal two-thirds a smooth, triangular, flattened area which is covered in the fresh state, by the tendons of the Extensor muscles. This surface is bounded by two lines, which commence in small tubercles situated on either side of the digital extremity, and, passing upward, converge and meet some distance above the center of the bone and form a ridge which runs along the rest of the dorsal surface to the carpal extremity. This ridge separates two sloping surfaces for the attachment of the Interossei dorsales. To the tubercles on the digital extremities are attached the collateral ligaments of the metacarpophalangeal joints.

The **Base** or **Carpal Extremity** (*basis*) is of a cuboidal form, and broader behind than in front: it articulates with the carpus, and with the adjoining metacarpal bones; its **dorsal** and **volar surfaces** are rough, for the attachment of ligaments.

The **Head** or **Digital Extremity** (*capitulum*) presents an oblong surface markedly convex from before backward, less so transversely, and flattened from side to side; it articulates with the proximal phalanx. It is broader, and extends farther upward, on the volar than on the dorsal aspect, and is longer in the antero-posterior than in the transverse diameter. On either side of the head is a tubercle for the attachment of the collateral ligament of the metacarpophalangeal joint. The **dorsal surface,** broad and flat, supports the Extensor tendons;

---

3 Henry Gray, Anatomy of the Human Body, 1918. With permission of Bartleby.com

the **volar surface** is grooved in the middle line for the passage of the Flexor tendons, and marked on either side by an articular eminence continuous with the terminal articular surface.

Characteristics of the Individual Metacarpal Bones.—The First Metacarpal Bone (*os metacarpale I; metacarpal bone of the thumb*) (Fig. 229) is shorter and stouter than the others, diverges to a greater degree from the carpus, and its volar surface is directed toward the palm. The **body** is flattened and broad on its dorsal surface, and does not present the ridge which is found on the other metacarpal bones; its volar surface is concave from above downward. On its radial border is inserted the Opponens pollicis; its ulnar border gives origin to the lateral head of the first Interosseus dorsalis. The **base** presents a concavo-convex surface, for articulation with the greater multangular; it has no facets on its sides, but on its radial side is a tubercle for the insertion of the Abductor pollicis longus. The **head** is less convex than those of the other metacarpal bones, and is broader from side to side than from before backward. On its volar surface are two articular eminences, of which the lateral is the larger, for the two sesamoid bones in the tendons of the Flexor pollicis brevis.

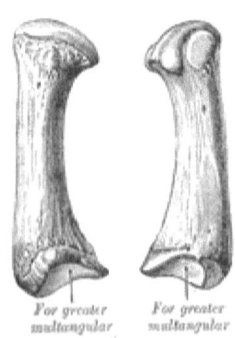

FIG. 229– *The first metacarpal. (Left.)*

The Second Metacarpal Bone (*os metacarpale II; metacarpal bone of the index finger*) (Fig. 230) is the longest, and its base the largest, of the four remaining bones. Its **base** is prolonged upward and medialward, forming a prominent ridge. It presents four articular facets: three on the upper surface and one on the ulnar side. Of the facets on the upper surface the intermediate is the largest and is concave from side to side, convex from before backward for articulation with the lesser multangular; the lateral is small, flat and oval for articulation with the greater multangular; the medial, on the summit of the ridge, is long and narrow for articulation with the capitate. The facet on the ulnar side articulates with the third metacarpal. The Extensor carpi radialis longus is inserted on the dorsal surface and the Flexor carpi radialis on the volar surface of the base.

The Third Metacarpal Bone (*os metacarpale III; metacarpal bone of the middle finger*) (Fig. 231) is a little smaller than the second. The dorsal aspect of its **base** presents on its radial side a pyramidal eminence, the **styloid process,** which extends upward behind the capitate; immediately distal to this is a rough surface for the attachment of the Extensor carpi radialis brevis. The carpal articular facet is concave behind, flat in front, and articulates with the capitate. On the radial side is a smooth, concave facet for articulation with the second metacarpal, and on the ulnar side two small oval facets for the fourth metacarpal.

The **Fourth Metacarpal Bone** (*os metacarpale IV; metacarpal bone of the ring finger*) (Fig. 232) is shorter and smaller than the third. The **base** is small and quadrilateral; its superior surface presents two facets, a large one medially for articulation with the hamate, and a small one laterally for the capitate. On the radial side are two oval facets, for articulation with the third metacarpal; and on the ulnar side a single concave facet, for the fifth metacarpal.

The **Fifth Metacarpal Bone** (*os metacarpale V; metacarpal bone of the little finger*) (Fig. 233) presents on its **base** one facet on its superior surface, which is concavo-convex and articulates with the hamate, and one on its radial side, which articulates with the fourth metacarpal. On its ulnar side is a prominent tubercle for the insertion of the tendon of the Extensor carpi ulnaris. The dorsal surface of the body is divided by an oblique ridge, which extends from near the ulnar side of the base to the radial side of the head. The lateral part of this surface serves for the attachment of the fourth Interosseus dorsalis; the medial part is smooth, triangular, and covered by the Extensor tendons of the little finger.

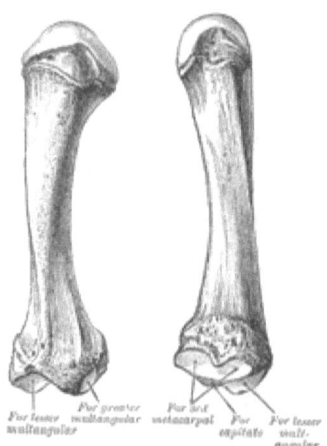

FIG. 230– The second metacarpal. (Left.)

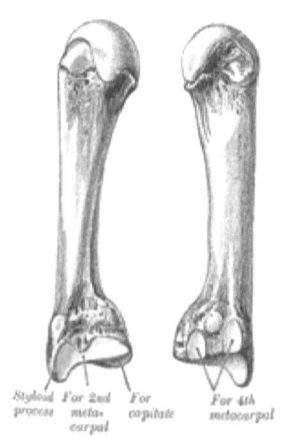

FIG. 231– The third metacarpal. (Left.)

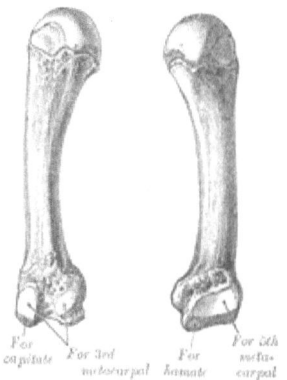

FIG. 232– The fourth metacarpal. (Left.)

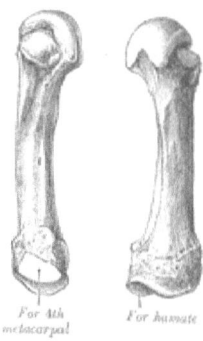

FIG. 233– The fifth metacarpal. (Left.)

PHALANGES

6B. 3. THE PHALANGES OF THE HAND

(PHALANGES DIGITORUM MANUS)

The **phalanges** are fourteen in number, three for each finger, and two for the thumb. Each consists of a body and two extremities. The **body** tapers from above downward, is convex posteriorly, concave in front from above downward, flat from side to side; its sides are marked by rough which give attachment to the fibrous sheaths of the Flexor tendons.

The **proximal extremities** of the bones of the first row present oval, concave articular surfaces, broader from side to side than from before backward. The **proximal extremity** of each of the bones of the second and third rows presents a double concavity separated by a median ridge. The **distal extremities** are smaller than the proximal, and each ends in two condyles separated by a shallow groove; the articular surface extends farther on the volar than on the dorsal surface, a condition best marked in the bones of the first row.

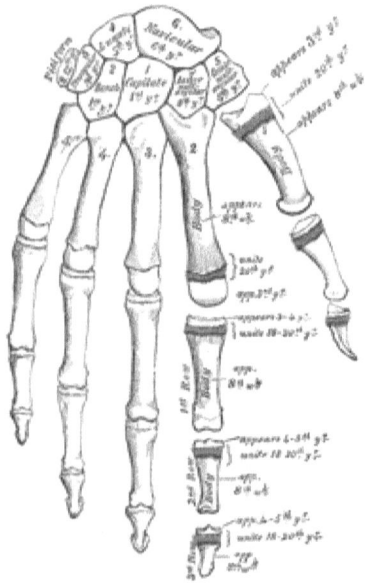

1F. The Muscles and Fasciæ of the Hand

The muscles of the hand are subdivided into three groups: (1) those of the thumb, which occupy the radial side and produce the **thenar eminence;** (2) those of the little finger, which occupy the ulnar side and give rise to the **hypothenar eminence;** (3) those in the middle of the palm and between the metacarpal bones.

Volar Carpal Ligament (*ligamentum carpi volare*).—The volar carpal ligament is the thickened band of antibrachial fascia which extends from the radius to the ulna over the Flexor tendons as they enter the wrist.

Transverse Carpal Ligament (*ligamentum carpi transversum; anterior annular ligament***) (Figs. 421, 422).**—The transverse carpal ligament is a strong, fibrous band, which arches over the carpus, converting the deep groove on the front of the carpal bones into a tunnel, through which the Flexor tendons of the digits and the median nerve pass. It is attached, medially, to the pisiform and the hamulus of the hamate bone; laterally, to the tuberosity of the navicular, and to the medial part of the volar surface and the ridge of the greater multangular. It is continuous, above, with the volar carpal ligament; and below, with the palmar aponeurosis. It is crossed by the ulnar vessels and nerve, and the cutaneous branches of the median and ulnar nerves. At its lateral end is the tendon of theFlexor carpi radialis, which lies in the groove on the greater multangular between the attachments of the ligament to the bone. On its volar surface the tendons of the Palmaris longus and Flexor carpi ulnaris are partly *inserted;* below, it gives origin to the short muscles of the thumb and little finger

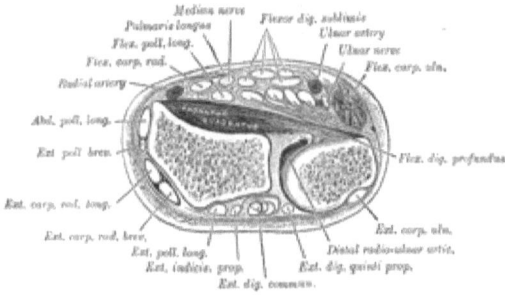

FIG. 421– Transverse section across distal ends of radius and ulna.

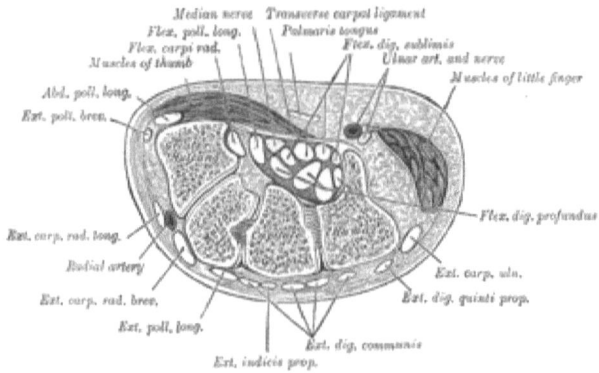

FIG. 422– Transverse section across the wrist and digits

The Mucous Sheaths of the Tendons on the Front of the Wrist.—
Two sheaths envelop the tendons as they pass beneath the transverse carpal ligament, one for the Flexores digitorum sublimis and profundus, the other for the Flexor pollicis longus (Fig. 423). They extend into the forearm for about 2.5 cm. above the transverse carpal ligament, and occasionally communicate with each other under the ligament. The sheath which surrounds the Flexores digitorum extends downward about half-way along the metacarpal bones, where it ends in blind diverticula around the tendons to the index, middle, and ring fingers. It is prolonged on the tendons to the little finger and usually communicates with the mucous sheath of these tendons. The sheath of the tendon of the Flexor pollicis longus is continued along the thumb as far as the insertion of the tendon.

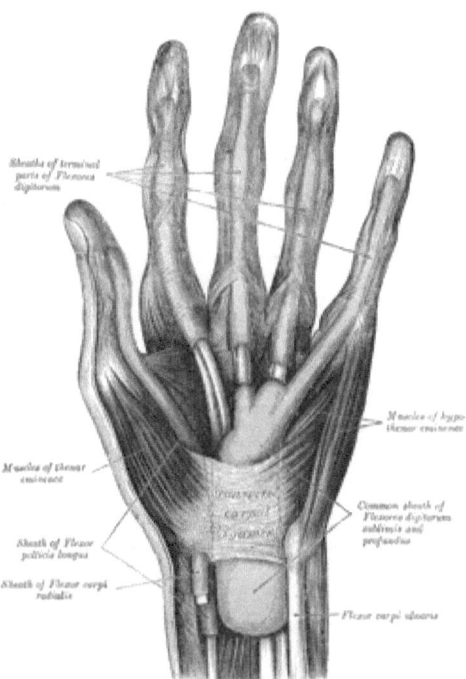

FIG. 423– The mucous sheaths of the tendons on the front of the wrist and digits.

Dorsal Carpal Ligament (*ligamentum carpi dorsale; posterior annular ligament*) (Figs. 421, 422).—The dorsal carpal ligament is a strong, fibrous band, extending obliquely downward and medialward across the back of the wrist, and consisting of part of the deep fascia of the back of the forearm, strengthened by the addition of some transverse fibers. It is attached, *medially,* to the styloid process of the ulna and to the triangular and pisiform bones; *laterally,* to the lateral margin of the radius; and, in its passage across the wrist, to the ridges on the dorsal surface of the radius.

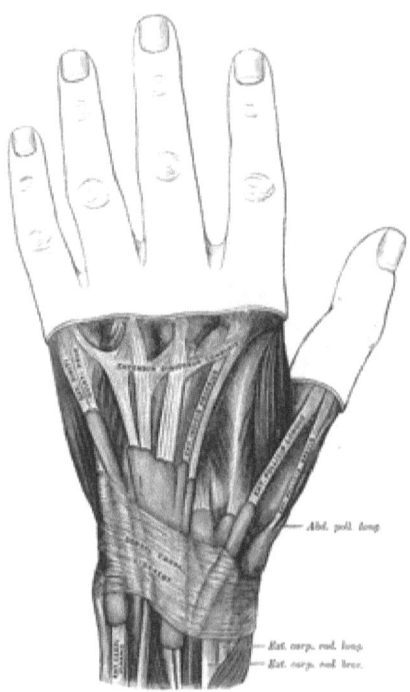

FIG. 424– The mucous sheaths of the tendons on the back of the wrist.

The Mucous Sheaths of the Tendons on the Back of the Wrist.—
Between the dorsal carpal ligament and the bones six compartments are
formed for the passage of tendons, each compartment having a separate
mucous sheath. One is found in each of the following positions (Fig.
424): (1) on the lateral side of the styloid process, for the tendons of the
Abductor pollicis longus and Extensor pollicis brevis; (2) behind the
styloid process, for the tendons of the Extensores carpi radialis longus
and brevis; (3) about the middle of the dorsal surface of the radius, for
the tendon of the Extensor pollicis longus; (4) to the medial side of
the latter, for the tendons of the Extensor digitorum communis and
Extensor indicis proprius; (5) opposite the interval between the radius
and ulna, for the Extensor digiti quinti proprius; (6) between the head
and styloid process of the ulna, for the tendon of the Extensor carpi
ulnaris. The sheaths lining these compartments extends from above
the dorsal carpal ligament; those for the tendons of Abductor pollicis
longus, Extensor brevis pollicis, Extensores carpi radialis, and Extensor

carpi ulnaris stop immediately proximal to the bases of the metacarpal bones, while the sheaths for Extensor communis digitorum, Extensor indicis proprius, and Extensor digiti quinti proprius are prolonged to the junction of the proximal and intermediate thirds of the metacarpus.

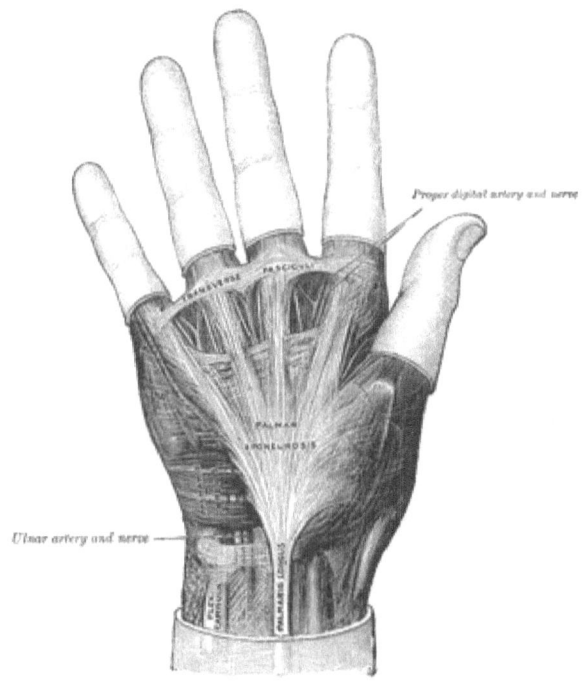

FIG. 425– The palmar aponeurosis.

Palmar Aponeurosis (*aponeurosis palmaris; palmar fascia*) (Fig. 425).—The palmar aponeurosis invests the muscles of the palm, and consists of central, lateral, and medial portions.

The **central portion** occupies the middle of the palm, is triangular in shape, and of great strength and thickness. Its apex is continuous with the lower margin of the transverse carpal ligament, and receives the expanded tendon of the Palmaris longus. Its base divides below into four slips, one for each finger. Each slip gives off superficial fibers to the skin of the palm and finger, those to the palm joining the skin at the furrow corresponding to the metacarpophalangeal articulations, and those to the fingers passing into the skin at the transverse fold at the bases of the fingers. The deeper part of each slip subdivides into two processes, which are inserted into the fibrous sheaths of the Flexor tendons. From the sides of these processes offsets are attached to the transverse metacarpal ligament. By this arrangement short channels are formed on the front of the heads of the metacarpal bones; through these the Flexor tendons pass. The intervals between the four slips transmit the digital vessels and nerves, and the tendons of the Lumbricales. At the points of division into the slips mentioned, numerous strong, transverse fasciculi bind the separate processes together. The central part of the palmar aponeurosis is intimately bound to the integument by dense fibroareolar tissue forming the superficial palmar fascia, and gives origin by its medial margin to the Palmaris brevis. It covers the superficial volar arch, the tendons of the Flexor muscles, and the branches of the median and ulnar nerves; and on either side it gives off a septum, which is continuous with the interosseous aponeurosis, and separates the intermediate from the collateral groups of muscles.

The **lateral** and **medial portions** of the palmar aponeurosis are thin, fibrous layers, which cover, on the radial side, the muscles of the ball of the thumb, and, on the ulnar side, the muscles of the little finger; they are continuous with the central portion and with the fascia on the dorsum of the hand.

The **Superficial Transverse Ligament of the Fingers** is a thin band of transverse fasciculi (Fig. 425); it stretches across the roots of the four fingers, and is closely attached to the skin of the clefts, and medially to the fifth metacarpal bone, forming a sort of rudimentary web. Beneath it the digital vessels and nerves pass to their destinations.

1. The Lateral Volar Muscles (Figs. 426, 427)

Abductor pollicis brevis.   Flexor pollicis brevis.

Opponens pollicis.   Adductor pollicis (obliquus).

Adductor pollicis (transversus).

The **Abductor pollicis brevis** (*Abductor pollicis*) is a thin, flat muscle, placed immediately beneath the integument. It *arises* from the transverse carpal ligament, the tuberosity of the navicular, and the ridge of the greater multangular, frequently by two distinct slips. Running lateralward and downward, it is *inserted* by a thin, flat tendon into the radial side of the base of the first phalanx of the thumb and the capsule of the metacarpophalangeal articulation.

The **Opponens pollicis** is a small, triangular muscle, placed beneath the preceding. It *arises* from the ridge on the greater multangular and from the transverse carpal ligament, passes downward and lateralward, and is *inserted* into the whole length of the metacarpal bone of the thumb on its radial side.

The **Flexor pollicis brevis** consists of two portions, lateral and medial. The **lateral** and more **superficial portion** *arises* from the lower border of the transverse carpal ligament and the lower part of the ridge on the greater multangular bone; it passes along the radial side of the tendon of the Flexor pollicis longus, and, becoming tendinous, is *inserted* into the radial side of the base of the first phalanx of the thumb; in its tendon of insertion there is a sesamoid bone. The **medial** and **deeper portion** of the muscle is very small, and *arises* from the ulnar side of the first metacarpal bone between the Adductor pollicis (obliquus) and the lateral head of the first Interosseous dorsalis, and is *inserted* into the ulnar side of the base of the first phalanx with the Adductor pollicis (obliquus). The medial part of the Flexor brevis pollicis is sometimes described as the **first Interosseous volaris.**

The **Adductor pollicis (obliquus)** (*Adductor obliquus pollicis*) *arises* by several slips from the capitate bone, the bases of the second and third metacarpals, the intercarpal ligaments, and the sheath of the tendon of the Flexor carpi radialis. From this origin the greater number of fibers pass obliquely downward and converge to a tendon, which, uniting with the tendons of the medial portion of the Flexor pollicis brevis and the transverse part of the Adductor, is *inserted* into the ulnar side of the base of the first phalanx of the thumb, a sesamoid bone being present in the tendon. A considerable fasciculus, however, passes more obliquely beneath the tendon of the Flexor pollicis longus to join the lateral portion of the Flexor brevis and the Abductor pollicis brevis.

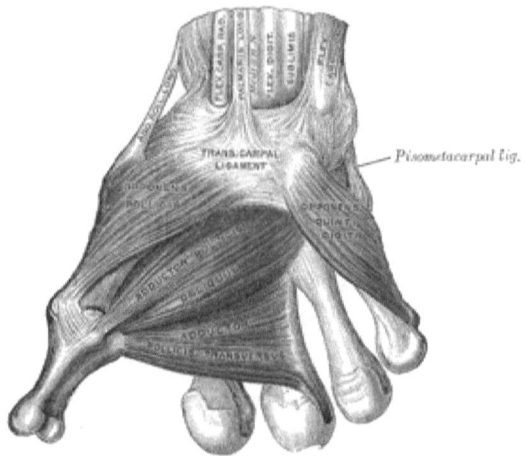

FIG. 426– The muscles of the thumb

The **Adductor pollicis (transversus)** (*Adductor transversus pollicis*) (Fig. 426) is the most deeply seated of this group of muscles. It is of a triangular form arising by a broad base from the lower two-thirds of the volar surface of the third metacarpal bone; the fibers converge, to be *inserted* with the medial part of the Flexor pollicis brevis and the Adductor pollicis (obliquus) into the ulnar side of the base of the first phalanx of the thumb.

Variations.—The Abductor pollicis brevis is often divided into an outer and an inner part; accessory slips from the tendon of the Abductor pollicis longus or Palmaris longus, more rarely from the Extensor carpi radialis longus, from the styloid process or Opponens pollicis or from the skin over the thenar eminence. The deep head of the Flexor pollicis brevis may be absent or enlarged. The two adductors vary in their relative extent and in the closeness of their connection. The Adductor obliquus may receive a slip from the transverse metacarpal ligament.

Nerves.—The Abductor brevis, Opponens, and lateral head of the Flexor pollicis brevis are supplied by the sixth and seventh cervical nerves through the median nerve; the medial head of the Flexor brevis, and the Adductor, by the eighth cervical through the ulnar nerve.

Actions.—The Abductor pollicis brevis draws the thumb forward in a plane at right angles to that of the palm of the hand. The Adductor pollicis is the opponent of this muscle, and approximates the thumb to the palm. The Opponens pollicis flexes the metacarpal bone, *i. e.,* draws it medialward over the palm; the Flexor pollicis brevis flexes and adducts the proximal phalanx.

2. The Medial Volar Muscles (Figs. 426, 427)

Palmaris brevis. Flexor digiti quinti brevis.

Abductor digiti quinti. Opponens digiti quinti.

The **Palmaris brevis** is a thin, quadrilateral muscle, placed beneath the integument of the ulnar side of the hand. It *arises* by tendinous fasciculi from the transverse carpal ligament and palmar aponeurosis; the fleshy fibers are inserted into the skin on the ulnar border of the palm of the hand.

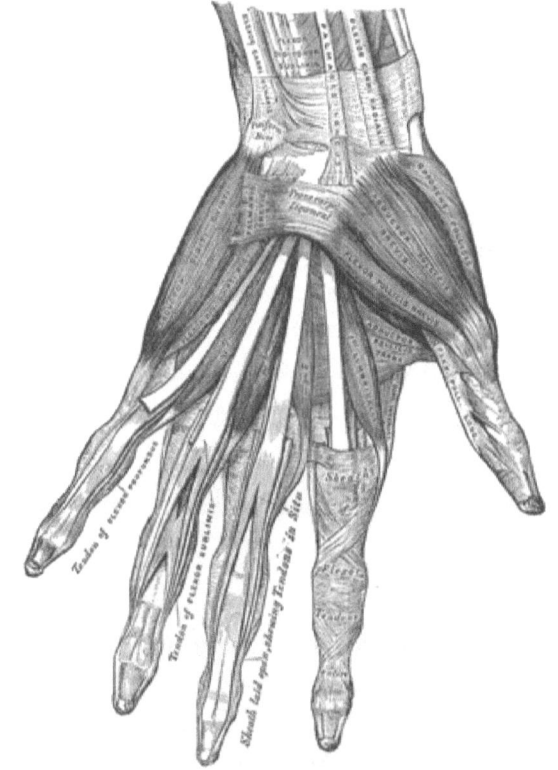

FIG. 427– The muscles of the left hand. Palmar surface

The **Abductor digiti quinti** (*Abductor minimi digiti*) is situated on the ulnar border of the palm of the hand. It *arises* from the pisiform bone and from the tendon of the Flexor carpi ulnaris, and ends in a flat tendon, which divides into two slips; one is *inserted* into the ulnar side of the base of the first phalanx of the little finger; the other into the ulnar border of the aponeurosis of the Extensor digiti quinti proprius.

The **Flexor digiti quinti brevis** (*Flexor brevis minimi digiti*) lies on the same plane as the preceding muscle, on its radial side. It *arises* from the convex surface of the hamulus of the hamate bone, and the volar surface of the transverse carpal ligament, and is *inserted* into the ulnar side of the base of the first phalanx of the little finger. It is separated from the Abductor, at its origin, by the deep branches of the ulnar artery and nerve. This muscle is sometimes wanting; the Abductor is then, usually, of large size.

The **Opponens digiti quinti** (*Opponens minimi digiti*) (Fig. 426) is of a triangular form, and placed immediately beneath the preceding muscles. It *arises* from the convexity of the hamulus of the hamate bone, and contiguous portion of the transverse carpal ligament; it is inserted into the whole length of the metacarpal bone of the little finger, along its ulnar margin.

Variations.—The Palmaris brevis varies greatly in size. The Abductor digiti quinti may be divided into two or three slips or united with the Flexor digiti quinti brevis. Accessory head from the tendon of the Flexor carpi ulnaris, the transverse carpal ligament, the fascia of the forearm or the tendon of the Palmaris longus. A portion of the muscle may insert into the metacarpal, or separate slips the *Pisimetacarpus, Pisiuncinatus* or the *Pisiannularis* muscle may exist.

Nerves.—All the muscles of this group are supplied by the eighth cervical nerve through the ulnar nerve.

Actions.—The Abductor and Flexor digiti quinti brevis abduct the little finger from the ring finger and assist in flexing the proximal phalanx. The Opponens digiti quinti draws forward the fifth metacarpal bone, so as to deepen the hollow of the palm. The Palmaris brevis corrugates the skin on the ulnar side of the palm.

3. The Intermediate Muscles

Lumbricales.   Interossei.

The **Lumbricales** (Fig. 427) are four small fleshy fasciculi, associated with the tendons of the Flexor digitorum profundus. The first and second *arise* from the radial sides and volar surfaces of the tendons of the index and middle fingers respectively; the third, from the contiguous sides of the tendons of the middle and ring fingers; and the fourth, from the contiguous sides of the tendons of the ring and little fingers. Each passes to the radial side of the corresponding finger, and opposite the metacarpophalangeal articulation is *inserted* into the tendinous expansion of the Extensor digitorum communis covering the dorsal aspect of the finger.

Variations.—The Lumbricales vary in number from two to five or six and there is considerable variation in insertions.

The **Interossei** (Figs. 428, 429) are so named from occupying the intervals between the metacarpal bones, and are divided into two sets, a dorsal and a volar.

The **Interossei dorsales** (*Dorsal interossei*) are *four* in number, and occupy the intervals between the metacarpal bones. They are bipenniform muscles, each *arising* by two heads from the adjacent sides of the metacarpal bones, but more extensively from the metacarpal bone of the finger into which the muscle is inserted. They are inserted into the bases of the first phalanges and into the aponeuroses of the tendons of the Extensor digitorum communis. Between the double origin of each of these muscles is a narrow triangular interval; through the first of these the radial artery passes; through each of the other three a perforating branch from the deep volar arch is transmitted.

The **first** or **Abductor indicis** is larger than the others. It is flat, triangular in form, and *arises* by two heads, separated by a fibrous arch for the passage of the radial artery from the dorsum to the palm of the hand. The lateral head *arises* from the proximal half of the ulnar border of the first metacarpal bone; the medial head, from almost the entire length of the radial border of the second metacarpal bone; the tendon is inserted into the radial side of the index finger. The **second** and **third** are inserted into the middle finger, the former into its radial,

27

the latter into its ulnar side. The **fourth** is inserted into the ulnar side of the ring finger.

The **Interossei volares** (*Palmar interossei*), three in number, are smaller than the Interossei dorsales, and placed upon the volar surfaces of the metacarpal bones, rather than between them. Each *arises* from the entire length of the metacarpal bone of one finger, and is *inserted* into the side of the base of the first phalanx and aponeurotic expansion of the Extensor communis tendon to the same finger.

The **first** *arises* from the ulnar side of the second metacarpal bone, and is *inserted* into the same side of the first phalanx of the index finger. The **second** *arises* from the radial side of the fourth metacarpal bone, and is *inserted* into the same side of the ring finger. The **third** *arises* from the radial side of the fifth metacarpal bone, and is *inserted* into the same side of the little finger. From this account it may be seen that each finger is provided with two Interossei, with the exception of the little finger, in which the Abductor takes the place of one of the pair.

As already mentioned, the medial head of the Flexor pollicis brevis is sometimes described as the **Interosseus volaris primus.**

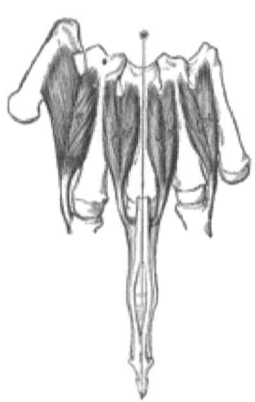

FIG. 428– The Interossei dorsales of left hand.

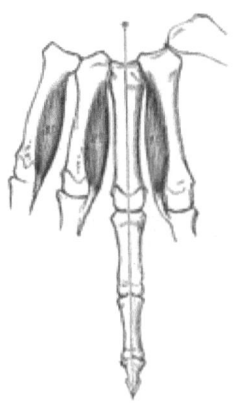

FIG. 429– The Interossei volares of left hand.

Actions.—The Interossei volares adduct the fingers to an imaginary line drawn longitudinally through the center of the middle finger; and the Interossei dorsales abduct the fingers from that line. In addition to this the Interossei, in conjunction with the Lumbricales, flex the first phalanges at the metacarpophalangeal joints, and extend the second and third phalanges in consequence of their insertions into the expansions of the Extensor tendons. The Extensor digitorum communis is believed to act almost entirely on the first phalanges.

ART

In the 1500s, Michelangelo painted the ceiling of the Sistine Chapel at the Vatican. In one of the most famous pieces of art in the world, Michelangelo portrays a scene from *Genesis* in which Adam and G-d are shown with their iconic fingers about to touch, symbolizing the transfer of life from G-d to Adam.

Other famous paintings in which the index finger plays a major role are Leonardo da Vinci's "John the Baptist;" and Raphael's "The School of Athens."

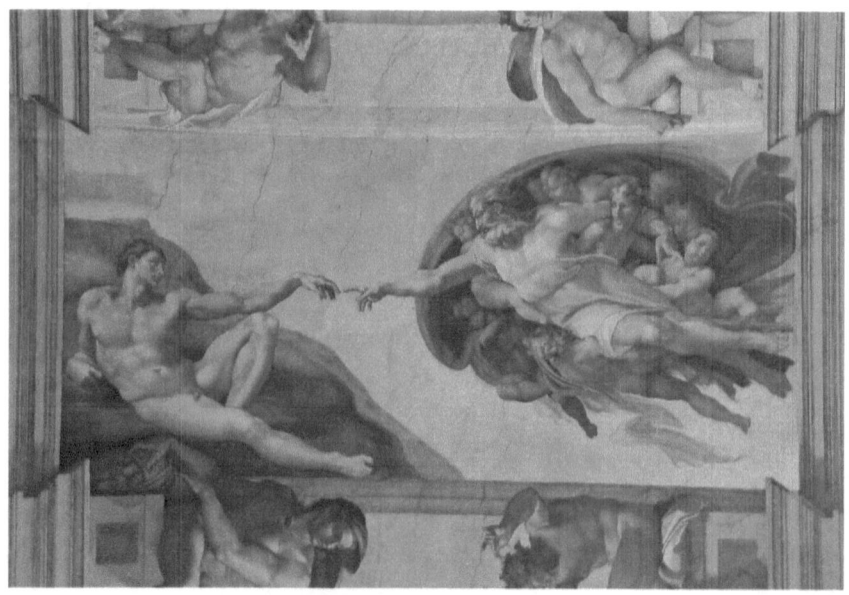

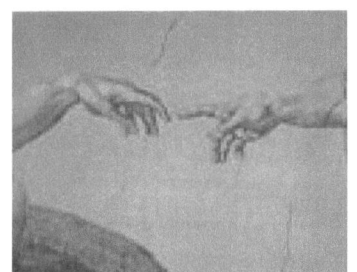

Sistine Chapel,
Michelangelo

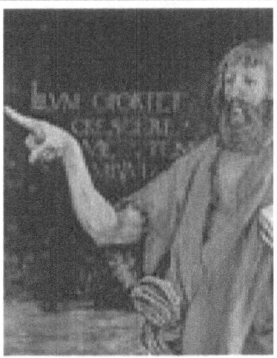

Isenheim Altarpiece,
John the Baptist

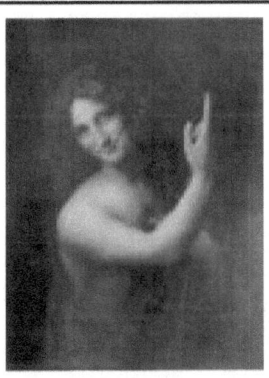

John the Baptist,
Leonardo da Vinci

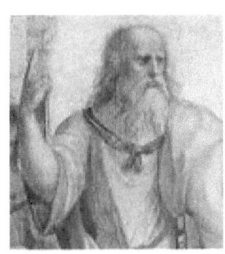

The School of Athens,
Raphael

CLICHÉ'S, IDIOMS, EPONYMS, TERMS, AND SLANG

A pinky promise (also known as a pinky swear)	It is made when a person wraps one of their pinky fingers around the other person's pinky and makes a promise. Traditionally, it's considered binding; the idea was originally that the person who breaks the promise must cut off his pinky finger.
All thumbs	A descriptive term meaning an awkward or clumsy person. Lacking physical coordination, skill, or grace.
Anatomical snuff box	It is a triangular depression formed on the radial aspect of the wrist when the thumb is extended and abducted. It is shaped by the arrangement of the extensor pollicis longus and the extensor pollicis brevis and abductor pollicis longus tendons.
Anti-thumb	Refers to the little finger.

Ape hand	A deformity in which the thumb is extended and the hand flattened. Ape hand is caused by atrophy of the muscles, often seen in progressive spinal muscular atrophy or lesions of the median and ulnar nerve.
Apollo finger	In palmistry, the ring finger and the mound below it.
Arachnodactyly	A condition with abnormally long and slender fingers. See Marfans syndrome.
Baby finger	A term for the little finger.
Baseball finger	See mallet finger.
Benediction sign	See Bishop's hand.
Bennett's fracture	An intra-articular fracture-subluxation of the 1st metacarpal.
Bishop's hand	A low ulna nerve palsy that causes clawing of the ring and little fingers, that results in the appearance of the hand, as in the sign of benediction.
Black thumb	The innate inability to make plants grow. A gardener who kills plants. Opposite of green thumb.
Blackberry thumb	A catch-all phrase that describes a repetitive stress injury of the thumb as a result of overusing small gadget keypads.

Bouchard's nodes	A firm, non tender cartilaginous and bony enlargement of the proximal interphalangeal joints of a finger, as in arthritis. Contrast with Heberden's nodes.
Boutonniere's finger	A deformity of the finger that results from disruption or attenuation of the central slip of the extensor apparatus of a finger. As a result, the lateral bands subluxate volarward, and the finger assumes a position of flexion at the proximal interphalangeal joint and hyperextension of the distal phalangeal joint. Contrast with Swan neck deformity.
Boxer's fracture	A common name for a fracture of the neck of the 5th metacarpal, usually associated with volar displacement of the metacarpal neck.
Camptodactyly	literally means "bent finger" in Greek. It is a congenital condition in which the little finger is held in a fixed flexion position at an interphalangeal joint.
Chisanbop	An abacus-like finger counting method.
Clinodactyly	A congenital condition in which the little finger is curved towards the ring finger.
Clubbed thumb	Term used to describe genetic or acquired clubbing of one or both thumbs.

Clubbing of the fingers	bulbous enlargement of the distal portion of the fingers; early sign of an underlying disease.
Coach's finger	Dorsal dislocation of one of the proximal interphalangeal joints.
Dactylonomy	The art of counting along one's fingers.
Digitus annularis	The ring finger in Latin.
Digitus II	The index finger.
Digitus impudicus	The impudent finger. A well-known obscene hand gesture made by extending the middle finger of the hand while bending the other fingers into the palm, with numerous alternative names.
Digitus medicinalis	The ring finger in Latin.
Digitus medio proximus	The ring finger in Latin.
Digitus secundus	The index finger.
Felon finger	An abscess of the distal finger where the pulp is divided into many fibrous septa. Also called Whitlow.
Finger	Any of the terminal members of the hand. Each person normal has five fingers on each hand. A fluid measure in alcoholic beverages.
Finger binary	A system for counting and displaying binary numbers on the fingers and thumbs of one or more hands.

Finger food	Food that is normally eaten without utensils (e.g. peanuts).
Finger in every pie	A phrase indicating that a person is involved in numerous activities concurrently. It usually has a negative connotation and implies that untruthful behavior is involved. It originated as a reference to someone eating many pies in a kitchen.
Finger lengths	An idea that finger lengths and finger length ratios have predictive qualities regarding intellectual abilities, physical attributes, and disease potentialities.
Finger lickin' good	A trademark of the KFC Corporation referring to their tasty chicken products.
Finger naming	A phrase that is used when an individual implicates or accuses another or others of some illicit activity or crime.
Finger Pointing	The act of blaming someone for something; the imputation of blame.
Finger on the pulse	This phrase means that a person is conscious of the most up-to-date events and information, therefore their heart rate is always active and can be checked by placing the fingertips on the pulse.
Finger protocol	The use of computer networking to obtain information on someone's status.

Finger puppet	Type of toy used to entertain children as different characters are created by use of puppets on the fingers. Can be made out of various materials.
Finger trouble	A phrase used to describe a mistake made by pushing an incorrect button on an electronic object.
Finger wagging	The act of waving the finger from side to side. Usually expresses the word "No". An admonitory gesture.
Fingering	The positioning of fingers when playing a musical instrument. A sexual act.
Fingers in the till (have your)	To steal money from the place where you work, usually from a shop.
Fingers were made before forks	A phrase justifying that it is acceptable to eat using one's fingers in place of a fork, since people were consuming food prior to the invention of forks.
Fish fingers	A type of food.
Flipping someone off	A well-known obscene hand gesture made by extending the middle finger of the hand while bending the other fingers into the palm, with numerous alternative names.
Forefinger	A term for the index finger.
Gamekeeper's thumb	A rupture of the ulnar collateral ligament of the metacarpophalangeal joint of the thumb.

Giving someone the finger	A well-known obscene hand gesture made by extending the middle finger of the hand while bending the other fingers into the palm, with numerous alternative names.
Green thumb	The ability to make plants grow. An innate ability to make plants grow. Natural talent for growing plants. Opposite of black thumb.
Heberden's nodes	A cartilaginous and bony enlargement at the distal interphalangeal joint of a finger, characteristic of osteoarthritis. Contrast with Bouchard's nodes.
Hypothenar muscles	The abductor digiti minimus, flexor digiti minimi, and opponens digiti minimi muscles.
Hypothenar space	The anatomic compartment on the ulnar side of the palm that contains the hypothenar muscles.
Index finger	The finger next to the thumb. Forefinger. trigger finger. digitus secundus. digitus II. Jupiter finger.
Jammed finger	A diffusely painful and swollen proximal interphalangeal joint of a digit, resulting from a sudden, longitudinally directed force on the extended proximal interphalangeal joint.
Jupiter finger	In palmistry, the index finger and the mound below it.

Keep your fingers crossed	A phrase meaning to hope and wish for the best, because they form a rough crucifix. From "Random House Dictionary of Popular Proverbs and Sayings" by Gregory Y. Titelman: "Hope for success. The saying derives from the superstition that bad luck may be averted by making the sign of the cross. Originated in the 1920s."
Little finger	The finger farthest from the thumb. Also called the pinky or baby finger. Latin: digitus minimus manus, digitus quintus, digitus V. Anti-thumb.
Kirner Deformity	Deviated phalanx of the little finger. Also known as dystelephalangy. Involves a bowing of the distal phalanx making it appear hooked.
Magical finger	The ring finger. Some cultures associate this finger to magical rings.

Mallet finger	A deformity of the finger in which the distal interphalangeal joint has an extension lag; this results from a disruption of the extensor tendon mechanism at or near its site of insertion into the distal phalanx. The patient can passively (but not actively) extend the distal phalanx at the distal interphalangeal joint. The injury is caused by a sharp blow on the end of the finger, as when struck by a baseball. Hence, its popular name, baseball finger.
Mercury finger	In palmistry, the little finger and the mound below it.
Midas finger (also known as Midas touch)	Named for the Greek mythological King Midas, whose touch turned everything to gold. In its modern usage, refers to someone who has an aptitude for making money.
Middle finger	The finger between the index and ring fingers. Also called the impudent finger.
Nameless Finger	The ring finger. It is called the nameless finger in various cultures.
Paronychium	Infection of the nail bed.
Pinkie	The little finger in Scottish English. In American English, pinky.

Pinky	The little finger in American English. It originates from the Dutch word *pink*, meaning little finger. Also called the anti-thumb, baby finger, and in Latin, digitus minimus manus, digitus quintus, digitus V.
Pinky swear (also known as pinky promise)	See pinky promise.
Pointer finger	The index finger.
Poland's Syndrome	A rare birth defect characterized by underdevelopment or absence of the pectoralis chest muscle on one side of the body on the same side (ipsilateral) associated with the webbing of the fingers (syndactyly).
Polydactyly	An excess of five digits on the hand; usually see six digits per hand, but seven or eight also occurs. It is the second most common congenital deformity involving the hand. Occurs in about every 1 of 3000 in the white population but is much more frequent in the black population (1 in 300).
Ring finger	The finger next to the little finger. Also called digitus medicinalis, digitus annularis, digitus quartus, or digitus IV. Wedding ring finger. Nameless finger. In Palmistry, the Apollo finger.

Rock, Paper, Scissors	A popular children's game involving both the hands and fingers.
Rule of thumb	This phrase originated from an old English law which said a man could not hit his wife with anything wider than his thumb.
Saturn finger	In palmistry, the middle finger and the mound below it.
Shooting a bird	A well known obscene hand gesture made by extending the middle finger of the hand while bending the other fingers into the palm.
Skier's thumb	A condition characterized by injuries to the thumb, especially the ulnar collateral ligament. See Gamekeeper's thumb.
Slip through one's fingers	Allowing an opportunity to pass you by.
Sucking thumb	A body language sign of regressive behavior, as in a return to childhood and breast feeding. This may indicate timidity and feelings of inferiority.
Swan neck deformity	A finger deformity involving flexion of the distal interphalangeal joint and hyperextension of the proximal interphalangeal joint. Contrast with Boutonniere deformity.
Syndactyly	A union of two or more digits that occur in humans as a familial anomaly marked by the webbing of two or more fingers or toes. It is the most common congenital deformity involving the hand.

The bird	A well-known obscene hand gesture made by extending the middle finger of the hand while bending the other fingers into the palm.
The Finger	A well known obscene hand gesture made by extending the middle finger of the hand while bending the other fingers into the palm.
The Medical finger	The ring finger. Some cultures named this finger after its supposed magical powers. In English, it's called the leech finger.
The Nameless finger	The ring finger. Many cultures avoided the use of a powerful entity and thus called it the nameless finger.
Thenar	Relating to, involving, or constituting the ball of the thumb or the intrinsic musculature of the thumb.
Thenar eminence	The prominent fleshy area of the palm of the hand, overlying the first metacarpal, whose bulk is formed by the thenar muscles.
Thenar muscles	The intrinsic muscles of the thumb that give prominence to the thenar eminence. They are the abductor pollicis brevis, the opponens pollicis, and the flexor pollicis brevis muscles.

Thumb	The short thick digit of the human hand, next to the index finger and opposable to each of the other fingers. Also called pollex. The part of a glove or mitten that provides a covering for the thumb.
Thumb a lift	This phrase refers to the event of attempting to get a ride from oncoming traffic by pointing your thumb in the target direction of one's destination. Also known as hitchhiking.
Thumb index	The grooves and indentations in a book that are labeled for easier page referencing and used for divisions in a book.
Thumb one's nose	To place the thumb at one's nose and extend the fingers as a gesture of scorn, derision, or defiance. To express scorn or ridicule by or as if by placing the thumb on the nose and wiggling the fingers.
Thumb sucking	The act of putting the thumb in the mouth and rhythmically repeating sucking contact for a prolonged duration.
Thumb through	To flip the pages of (a book or magazine) in order to glance at the contents. Peruse.
Thumb twiddling	Activity done by the hands in which the fingers interlock and the thumbs circle around a common point.

Thumb wrestling	A popular children's game that involves two opponents and their thumbs.
Thumbing	Synonym for hitchhiking. A finishing technique in pottery production. The act of typing on a small keyboard with thumbs.
Thumbnail	A small representation of a picture or graphic on a Web page, usually containing a hyperlink to a full-size version of the graphic. A miniature, low resolution version of an image or illustration.
Thumbs down	Activity used to show dislike or disapproval. In the Roman amphitheater the crowd reputedly used this signal to suggest to the emperor that a defeated gladiator be killed.
Thumbs up	Activity used to show acceptance or approval. In the Roman amphitheatre the crowd reputedly used this signal to suggest that a defeated gladiator be spared. In some Middle Eastern countries, this gesture is considered just as offensive as the middle finger. Several countries use this expression in saying, "Up yours, pal." Thumbs up when the hands are in a pocket is often a body language sign of confidence, relaxed and in control. In contrast to thumbs down.

To give the finger	This phrase means to raise the middle finger at someone as an obscene gesture.
Tom Thumb	1838-83, American entertainer, whose original name was Charles Sherwood Stratton. His career as General Tom Thumb began in 1842, when the showman P. T. Barnum gave him the title and arranged with the child's parents for his exhibition as a midget.
Trigger finger	A painful snapping and locking of the finger in marked flexion, caused by a nodular swelling and stenosis of the flexor tendon at the level of the metacarpo-phalangeal joint. On unclenching a fist, the affected finger at first remains bent. Then, overcoming the resistance, it suddenly straightens (triggers).
Trigger Thumb	A trigger finger affecting the thumb.
Under one's thumb Under the thumb	Under the influence or power of a person. Under the control of someone; subordinate to.
V-sign	Involves raising both the index and middle fingers into a 'V' shape. Means "Peace". Means "Victory". Used as a salute during the Hundred Years' War.

Vulcan salute	From the Star Trek television series. It is a symbol for "Live long and prosper." The hand figure is made by separating the hand into three parts: the thumb spread apart from the index and middle fingers; and then the ring and little fingers.
Wagging the finger	The act of waving the finger from side to side. Usually expresses the word "No". An admonitory gesture.
Webbed fingers	A congenital condition in which the adjacent fingers are abnormality connected by excess skin and subcutaneous tissue at their bases; syndactyly.
Whitlow	See felon.
Wrapped around your finger	To have authority or power over another individual.

DIGITUS MEDICINALIS – THE ETYMOLOGY OF THE NAME[4]

László A. Magyar

Ring finger is indicated in Latin by three names. It is either called «the finger proximal to the middle finger » (digitus medio proximus) or ring finger (digitus annularis) or medical finger (digitus medicinalis or medicus). This latter term can also be found in Greek. Whether the Latin or the Greek expression had occurred primarily can currently be decided only with difficulty.

The name digitus medicinalis has already aroused the attention of the antique authors, since it is not at all obvious what ring finger has to do with medicine. The only authentic ancient reference to the origins of the name can be found in Galen's *Eisagoge* which reads as follows: «...this is followed by the finger proximal to the middle one which is devoted to physicians (toiv iatroiv anakeimenov)... and was named after them (am autwn tounoma keklmrwmenov).

Two things can be concluded from Galen's sentence. On the one hand, that the medical finger is actually identical with the ring finger – some authors consider namely the middle finger as digitus medicinalis (6) and on the other hand, that the ring finger is somehow linked with medicine. But how is it linked? This question is going to be answered in the following.

---

4 Actes du Congr. Intern. d'Hist. de Med. XXXII., Antwerpen, 1990. 175-179.

Of the antique traditions associated with the ring finger, one of the most interesting example in this respect is a text from the work Attic Nights of Aulus Gellius, a contemporary of Galen: «According to our knowledge» – writes Gellius - «ancient Greeks wore their ring on the finger of their left hand proximal to the little finger. The Romans were assumed to wear their rings also there. Apion attributed it, in his books on Egypt, to the cause that Egyptians, when, according to their customs, cut and dissected the human body – this is called anatomy in Greek – detected a slim nerve, which, originating in the finger mentioned above proceeds and penetrates quite up to the human heart. There fore, it does not seem to be unjustified to adorn this finger in such a way, which, in view of the above, is related to the heart, the prince of the body.

Enlarging upon it, this tradition can otherwise also be found in the work *Saturnalia* of Macrobius in the 4th century. The data of Gellius should, however, be treated with some caution, partly because Apion's work mentioned by him has been lost and partly because it was not unanimously stated either by Macrobius or Gellius that the name digitus medicinalis should be associated with this tradition. They explain only the ring-wearing with the anatomical role of this finger.

In addition, there is no trace of the view entertained by Gellius in the preserved Egyptian medical texts, although in the text of Macrobius the Egyptian cultic importance of the ring finger is verified by other examples, too. Anyway, the records are supported by the fact that an important role was attributed by Egyptian – and Greek – thinking to the nerves or vessels proceeding from the heart solely because of the importance of the heart itself: the heart is often referred to as the centre of vitality and procreative power, and there is also clue – if not in the Egyptian but some other near-eastern traditions – that vital force originating in the heart can also be concentrated in the finger. In other places there are references of the association between the ring finger of the left hand, the procreative power and the principle of maternity.

An Egyptian conception actually existed or could at least have existed according to which a vessel ascends from the heart to the ring finger. However, the scientific explanations of Gellius and Macrobius – as already pointed out by Bachofen, too – are still not satisfactory and rather seem to be the rational explanation of a belief. Besides these languages its identical term occurs in the German (*Arzt-Finger*) and in the Hungarian (orvos ujj), in both cases probably a metaphrase of the Latin Expression. But what about the other languages?

In the European languages the ring finger could also have three names: it could be named after the ring worn on it (e.g. *annulaire, Ring-finger, anulare*) – this being the most widely used version, or its position or sequence is designated by its name (e.g. *third-finger, digitus medio proximus*), and finally, it can assume a cover name obscure in origin (e.g. *Gold-Finger, Herz-Finger, bezimennij palec*, etc.). Let us have a look into what is common in these types of name.

As regards the name ring finger, the ring is the most powerful, magic symbol, that of the aion-snake of eternity, the symbol of the intertwining of life and death: it can attach significance to any of our fingers. On the other hand, the ring finger is not always a typically ring-wearing finger, and so the function of wearing a ring is difficult to interpret. The question arises, namely whether the finger could wear the ring because it had from the outset been endowed with magic power, or just the other way round, it was endowed, with magic power because it wore a ring. (According to some explanations, we wear ring on this finger, because this is the most indispensable and most protected one: affording the maximum safety to the jewel. Anyway, it is probable that the name ring finger suggests a magic power also in itself.

The names of fingers according to their position on the hand can also be related to magic, since by the rules of magic thinking, generally the thing is marked by a number which is not advisable to address by its real name. It is also to be considered the this is the only finger designated by an ordinal number, perhaps just to keep away from its magic power.

The third type of name mentioned here, the cover name (e.g. *Gold-Finger, Herz-Finger, anonymous finger*, etc.), inspired by whatever ideas, refers also unanimously to magic power, the function of cover name is just to render this power harmless.

All this is mainly clear in case of the «anonymous finger », the *par excellence* cover name. This peculiar name has been strikingly widely used in the languages of the most varied origin. The ring finger is named «anonymous finger» among others also in Persian (*binàme*), in Sanskrit (*andman*), in Hungarian (*nevetlen ujj*), in Finnish (*nimeton sormi*), in

Turkish (*adsiz parmak*), in Tartar (*atsyz parmak*), in Buryat-Mongolian (*nereguy hurgan*), in Russian (*benzymennyi palets*), or in Bulgarian (*benzimen pryst*). The magic character of this name has already been pointed out by several authors.

It could be seen that almost all of the ring-finger names supported the magic power of the ring finger. It can thus be stated that these names, in spite of the seeming differences in them are related with each other, since all suggest a magic power. On the other hand, it can be assumed – and that's what I wanted to get at – that the name digitus medicinalis is no exception to this rule either.

There is ample linguistic evidence for the magic significance of the ring finger. Fingers in general are of magic importance. This magic power manifests in the healing ability, ring finger is of exceptional importance also in this respect. According to Hungarian beliefs, e.g. the ring finger is not only suitable for curing abscesses warts, inflammation, diphteria and other illnesses, but also for as an aphrodisiac, partly indirectly, and partly as a means of transmitting medicine, as well as with the help of blood withdrawn from it. All this is so not only in Hungarian lore, but e.g. in the German and Slavic too. It is also sure that these beliefs are adequately ancient, too, verified by the already cited text of Pliny, Macrobius and Gellius.

Before drawing conclusions, let us examine the name digitus medicinalis itself. The adjective medicinalis originates from the verb *medeor* (medico), the original meaning of which is not else than «to heal by magic ». The verb can be traced back to the stem *med* – this stem designates «middle» - that is how perhaps the original meaning of the word medicus, i.e. «mediator» (medium), a mediator between humans and the world of spirits (i.e. magician) can be interpreted. That this is not only a mere brain wave is proved not only by a line of Silius Italicus, naming magicians *medicum vulgus*, but also by series of linguistic parallels, too (e.g. in German the word *Arzt* has originally meant also magician, while the Greek iatros derives form *iaino* of similar connotations.

In conclusion, the following statements can be made: based on linguistic and ethnographic examples, it seems to be evident that the ring finger is a finger of magic power. It appears to be sure that the ring-finger names almost always indicate the magic power of the finger: in this respect, according to our assumption, the Latin *digitus medicinalis* is not an exception either, since according to its original meaning, it is more correct to translate this expression not as «medical» but as «magic» finger. So Galen was wrong this time: the ring finger received this peculiar name not from the physicians but from the most: ancient way of healing, i.e. magic. Consequently, in the name *digitus medicinalis* the ancient meaning of the word *medicinalis* can be detected, this being none else than «magic».

DREAM SYMBOLS - HANDS AND FINGERS[5]

We create so much with our hands. In dreams, they can symbolize physical, artistic and psychological abilities.

Through writing, we can record precious memories or create new stories. Through touching, we create security and love. Through everyday tasks, we create dinners and a clean environment. We operate vehicles, computers, washing machines and lawn mowers. We create the image that we want the world to see when we use our hands to apply makeup or arrange our hair. We might create art through painting, sculpture and music. As an extension of our personalities, we use our hands to express ourselves much in the same way we use our eyes. Hands can also hurt and destroy. All of these tasks integrate the physical, psychological and emotional.

Consider what activity your hands are engaged in within your dream. Their gestures will help you decipher the message from your unconscious and the feelings you need to express. For instance, joined hands may represent love, a union or a relationship. A fist represents anger or a threat of danger. A raised hand may represent a blessing. A palm may represent the future. Using your hands to create or destroy something may represent a new idea or a desire to make a change in your life.

Sigmund Freud maintained that fingers were phallic symbols in dreams. Fingers can represent agility or its opposite, an impaired

5   With permission of <u>Aisling Ireland</u>, editor, BellaOnline's <u>Dreams</u>

or complete lack of ability. Reflect upon whether you are feeling confident or incompetent.

Is the finger pointing at someone, something or toward a certain direction? Your unconscious may be trying to help you solve a problem. A finger pointing at you may symbolize self-blame, guilt or accusation. Take a look at whether you can connect this to a situation in waking life.

May all your dreams come true!

EMBRYOLOGY

1. The branch of biology that deals with the formation, early growth, and development of living organisms.
2. The embryonic structure or development of an organism.
3. The study of the embryo and its development from a single-celled zygote (fertilized ovum) to the establishment of form and shape (at which point, if it is an animal, it becomes a fetus).

The hand and fingers follow a typical embryological developmental pattern:

Week 3 fetal development

Embryogenesis of the upper extremity commences with formation of the upper-limb bud on the lateral wall of the embryo three weeks after fertilization.

In the third week of fetal life the arm bud develops from the fifth through eight myotomes, and is first observed as a swelling in the low cervical region.

Then, the digits first appear as five projecting thickenings from the end of the limb plate at three weeks of fetal age. (Ireland, 1976)[6]

Week 4 fetal development

During the fourth week of gestation, the hand plate emerges, partially rimmed by a digital plate.

6 Ireland, D.C.R.: Poland's syndrome. In The Journal of Bone & Joint Surgery.58:52-58, 1976.

Week 5 fetal development

At the fifth week mark the upper and lower limbs have formed and look like finlike appendages, pointing laterally.

During the fifth week, radial condensations of mesoderm within the digital plate form the fingers, or digital rays. The digital rays are separated by webs of interdigital tissue. Within the interdigital space, radial apoptotic zones form, and programmed cell death first indents the dorsal surface. The distal tips then separate, and programmed cell death carves out the interdigital space proximally toward the central carpal region. (Dao, 2004)[7]

Week 6 fetal development

By six weeks the intervening tissue has disappeared, leaving the web spaces. (Ireland, 1976)

At the sixth week mark the limbs curve anteriorly. The interdigital space has formed by the end of the sixth week, but the digits continue to elongate and develop ventral tactile pads and undergo phalangeal differentiation. (Dao, 2004)

Week 7 fetal development

At seven weeks the hand contains its complement of skeletal elements as cartilage, except for the distal row of phalanges which still are represented as masses of condensed mesechchyme. (Ireland, 1976)

Week 8 fetal development

Eight weeks after fertilization, embryogenesis is complete and all limb structures are present.

The majority of congenital anomalies of the upper extremity occur during this period of rapid limb development, from week 4 to week 8. For example:

---

7   Dao, K.: Surgical Treatment of Congenital Syndactyly of the Hand. In The Journal of the American Academy of Orthopaedic Surgeons. Vol 12, No 1, 2004.

Syndactyly is the webbing of the fingers. Advances in molecular biology have provided insight into the embryologic etiology of syndactyly. On a molecular level, the formation of separate and independent digits occurs via a complicated interaction between fibroblast growth factors (FGFs), sonic hedgehog protein, bone morphogenic proteins (BMPs), and homeobox transcription factors, with MSX2 the most important. These factors, in turn, are regulated by the apical ectodermal ridge (AER), which is known to have a critical role in determining digit identity and formation of the interdigital space.

Early in limb development, FGF-10 expression within the lateral plate mesoderm induces FGF-8 and FGF-4 expression in the distal ectoderm destined to become the AER. Subsequently, cooperative interaction between AER-generated FGFs and sonic hedgehog protein secreted from the zone of polarizing activity regulates BMP expression within the mesoderm, forming a gradient across the cranial-caudal axis (anterior-posterior axis) that provides positional cues for digit identity. (Dao, 2004)

Finger Body Language[8]

Pointer

A pointing finger indicates direction ("It's over there"). For a long distance, the finger may be pointed diagonally upwards, as if firing an arrow. The index finger is usually used, though the middle finger or even all fingers may be used.

The thumb may be used to point to something being as it is jerked over the shoulder.

Pointing at people is like using the prod and is often considered to be rude and threatening. Angry people tend to point more often, including at themselves (when they feel hurt or insulted) and at those who they feel are to blame.

Club

The wagging finger of admonition beats up and down as if striking the culprit. This can be with a stable hand and just a finger way. It may also be done with the whole arm, giving an exaggerated striking movement.

A more polite version points downwards as it beats out an important point, perhaps tapping on something like a table.

The forefinger held up and stationary means 'wait' (perhaps as a threat of being used as a club otherwise).

---

8   With permission of ChangingMinds.org

Prod

The finger prod can act like a stiletto knife, stabbing forward at the other person. This is usually the index finger, although the middle finger is sometimes used. This is often very threatening and felt as a personal attack.

The prod may also be used to prod downwards at an imaginary item in front. This is less threatening than pointing directly at the person.

The prod can also be made less threatening by bringing several fingers together and bending the fingers. A disguised form of this is the finger-and-thumb pinch, where an imaginary idea is delicately held and offered forward.

Plate

Fingers extended and closed join with the palm to form a plate. The plate holds symbolic things, such as ideas, often gently. The plate may be proffered forwards, offering the held item to others. For large things both hands may be held together.

Held under the chin, it presents the face as an object to be admired and is often used in flirting.

Cup

Fingers held together and curled upwards form a cup that can contain things more securely than the plate. Relaxed fingers form a loose cup, whilst tense fingers form a more closed cup. Two hands together form a big cup (to hold bigger things).

Cups may be used to plead for something to be given or offer something forward to others.

Pinch

Fingers pinched together hold something small and delicate. This may be finger and thumb or may involve more fingers (finger and thumb is less frequent as this forms an 'O' which can have many different meanings).

It may be used when saying 'you must grasp this idea'. Held out towards others it offers them the idea. Pushed down it holds the idea whilst beating out the key points.

Claw

Curved and separated fingers form a claw. With palm facing down, the claw may threaten to reach forward and grab, scratch or tear.

If the fingers are held loosely, the shape is more of an open cup and may thus hold something. Held downwards it may gently restrain.

Drumming

Drumming or tapping the fingers can indicate frustration, for example when another person is speaking and the person wants to interrupt. It may also mean that the person drumming wants to leave.

Non-verbal noise sends an audible interrupt signal to the other person. The louder the noise and faster the drumming, the greater the tension the person is feeling. Drumming with the nails makes an even louder noise and hence sends a more urgent signal.

Drumming can also indicate that the person is thinking, and that the frustration is with internal thoughts and perhaps that an easy solution cannot be found.

Rudeness

The middle finger pointing upwards says 'up yours' and symbolizes a penis. The little finger in this gesture indicates the other person has a small penis (this is sometimes used as a rude gesture from a woman to a man).

The first two fingers pointing upwards and with the palm towards the self says 'f**k off' (though curiously, with the palm facing the other person indicates peace).

The finger and thumb together forming a circle may symbolize the female genitalia (perhaps likening the other person to this). It can also indicate the anus. Moved up and down it may indicate male masturbation (implying the other person, a male, is unable to gain a female partner and thus has to masturbate to get sexual relief). Yet with little finger facing outwards it can also mean 'OK' or 'wonderful'.

The index and little finger pointing upwards as a gesture can say that the other man is a cuckold. It can also signify the 'evil eye'.

Thumb

Thumbs-up signals approval and agreement. Thumbs-down signals disapproval. Held sideways (and perhaps waggled) indicates uncertainty).

Roman amphitheater audiences reputedly used this signal to suggest to the emperor that a defeated gladiator be spared or killed.

Thumbs up when arms are crossed or a single hand is held across the chest is a subtle sign of approval. It can also be an invitation to others to show approval of what you are saying.

Thumbs sticking out when hands are in pockets is often a sign of confidence, feeling relaxed and in control. It can thus be both a sign of authority and also of friendliness.

Also...

Inspecting fingernails indicates boredom and disinterest.

Fluttering fingers may indicate uncertainty ('I'm not sure') or may be a small wave (for example being child-like, indicating 'I am not a threat' or 'protect me').

Fidgeting fingers may indicate boredom or tension.

Sucking fingers is a regressive return to childhood and breast feeding. This may well indicate timidity and feelings of inferiority.

FINGER COUNTING

Dactylonomy is the art of counting along one's fingers.

One of the many skills we learn in preschool is to count on our fingers.

Our ten fingers are useful tools in learning the base-ten numeral system, with the fingers used as representations for the numerical digits

Finger counting, however, is nothing new. Significantly, different systems flourished in many cultures, far more sophisticated than the one-by-one finger count taught today.

How fingers may have been used to count

By N.S.Gill, About.com[9]

Counting on one's fingers seems a natural way to compute numbers, but the Greco-Romans didn't just count "on" their fingers. They counted with their fingers and not to be quick and accurate with the finger symbols could be embarrassing.

Evidence, particularly from the Imperial Roman world, comes from archaeology and ancient writers. Archaeological evidence comes from tombs, mosaics, and tesserae (dice), which last show finger symbols on one side and Roman numerals on the other.

---

9 ©2008 by N.S. Gill (http://ancienthistory.about.com/od/abacus/qt/FingerNumbers.htm). Used with permission of About, Inc. which can be found online at www.about.com. All rights reserved

Burma P. Williams and Richard S. Williams, in their article "Finger Numbers in the Roman World and the Early Middle Ages," from *Isis*, Vol. 86, No. 4 (Dec. 1995), pp. 587-608, state that Quintilian said an orator would be considered uneducated were he hesitant in calculating or used the wrong gestures with his fingers while making a calculation. This shows that fingers were probably not just used to show numbers, but to perform operations like addition and subtraction on them. However, as the authors state, we don't know whether the ancients used their fingers merely to keep track of intermediate stages while making mental calculations or whether they used their fingers to actually perform the computations.

This finger number system appears to have been in used throughout the Greco-Roman world and well into the Middle Ages. That the Greeks used fingers for computations seems to be implicit in the Homeric term for counting, pempathai, which means to count by fives.

The article mentions a riddle (from Symphosius and Alcuin) which seems to show something about how counting was done: How can 7 from 8 equal 6? Since the number 8 was represented by lowering the little and ring finger of the left hand and the number 7 was represented by lowering just the little finger, if you start with the 8 -- i.e., little and ring finger lowered -- and then raise the little finger to subtract the 7, the ring finger remains lowered and that was the symbol for 6. Obviously, the wrong

Medieval Finger Counting

The merchants of Medieval Europe and the Middle East used a system of finger counting. They could do rapid calculations on their fingers and keep track of money during the bargaining process. This type of finger counting is a place value system. The digits in the ones place are represented on the little, ring, and middle fingers of the left hand.

FINGER BINARY[10]

Finger binary is a system for counting and displaying binary numbers on the fingers and thumbs of one or more hands. Binary is composed of 1's and 0's. It is possible to display all numbers from 0 through 1023 (2^{10}–1) if both hands are used.

The thumb represents the value 1, the index is double that, so it's 2, and the middle is double the index, so it's 4, etc. This is key to understanding and fluently counting in binary on your fingers.

Fingers are given the following values:

- Holding one's right hand as a fist = 0
- One's <u>thumb</u> = 1 = (2^{1-1})
- One's <u>index finger</u> = 2 = (2^{2-1})
- One's <u>middle finger</u> = 4 = (2^{3-1})
- One's <u>ring finger</u> = 8 = (2^{4-1})
- One's <u>little finger</u> = 16 = (2^{5-1})
- One's left hand little finger = 32 = (2^{6-1})
- One's left hand ring finger = 64 = (2^{7-1})
- One's left hand middle finger = 128 = (2^{8-1})
- One's left hand index finger = 256 = (2^{9-1})
- One's left hand thumb = 512 = (2^{10-1})

All of both hand's fingers = 1023 = (2^{11-1}–1) Any combination = the fingers that are up's number + all other fingers that are up's numbers

CHISANBOP

Chisanbop, an abacus-like finger counting method. The fingers on your right hand keep track of the ones, and your left hand keeps track of the tens. **Fingers are worth 1 (or 1 group of ten) and thumbs are worth five (or five groups of ten).**

---

10 From Wikepedia.org

Spread your fingers out above a flat surface. Keep your fingers straight. Fingers that are touching the surface are "activated" and keep track of the numbers. To count to ten, start with your right index finger (one), then the middle finger (two), ring finger (three), little(four). To get to five, you simultaneously touch down your thumb and lift all four fingers. That is five. Six is thumb and index finger, seven is thumb and index and middle finger, etc., up to nine.

Chinese Method

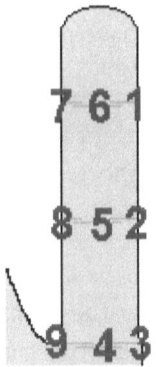

This is a Chinese method of counting to 100,000 on one hand. The little finger gives the units, as described above. The points marked are on the left, middle or right of the finger joints. The ring finger gives 10, 20, 30, 40, 50, 60, 70, 80 and 90 in a similar way. The middle finger covers the hundreds, again in a similar way. The index finger does the thousands, and the thumb does the ten thousands. The top of the thumb is 100,000.

FINGER LENGTH

Numerous articles and research projects discuss the idea that finger lengths and finger length ratios have predictive qualities.

During embryonic stages, a difference in the levels of hormone exposure results in a difference in the length of fingers. A higher level of prenatal testosterone exposure predicts a shorter index finger when compared to the ring finger length.

In women, the two fingers are usually almost equal in length, as measured from the crease nearest the palm to the fingertip. In males, the index finger is often slightly shorter than the ring finger. Whereas in females, the index finger is usually about the same size or somewhat longer than the ring finger.

A person's **finger-ratio is the index finger's length divided by the ring finger's length**. In men, the average **ratio** is 0.95. For women, 0.97

The following are various predictions that have been made using finger lengths:

- Aggression in men: A 2004 study by the University of Alberta shows that the shorter the index finger to ring finger ratio the more likely the male will be an aggressive adult.

- Athletic prowess: Studies have also found that a smaller index finger compared with the ring finger indicates a better athlete.

- <u>Autism:</u> Researchers have found that autistic children tended to have very low finger ratios.

- <u>Osteoarthritis:</u> A 2007 study by Zhang et al of the University of Nottingham, England found that the index to ring finger ratio is associated with osteoarthritis. Women who have a ring finger that is longer than the index finger have a greater risk of developing osteoarthritis in the knee.

- <u>SAT performance:</u> A 2007 study by Mark Brosnan of the University of Bath, England, have shown that a longer ring finger (a greater prenatal exposure to testosterone) suggests that the male will be better at math than literacy. For girls, a lower prenatal level of testosterone resulted in a smaller ring finger ratio to the index finger and these girls had higher SAT literacy scores.

- <u>Sexual Orientation:</u> Various studies have shown that finger length ratios may be a factor in sexual orientation.

FINGERNAILS

FINGERTIP ANATOMY[11]

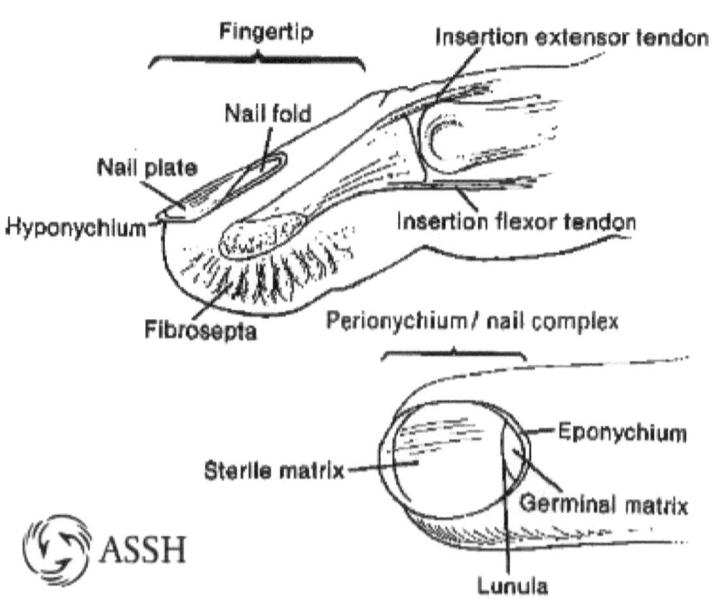

11 Images © 2002 American Society for Surgery of the Hand *Essentials of Hand Surgery*

The nails are specialized skin appendages derived from the epidermis. They grow from a germinal matrix located at the base of the distal phalanx just distal to the insertion of the extensor tendon to the hyponychium. Nails are made of protein, keratin, and sulfur.

Anatomy of the nail

- Cuticle (eponychium): The skin that folds over the nail

- Lunula: The white colored half moon at the nail bed

- Matrix: The area under the cuticle where nail growth occurs; it is very vascular, which accounts for the pink color. The entire nail matrix is in intimate contact with the periosteum of the distal phalanx

- Nail Bed: The soft, connective tissue under the nail

- Nail Folds (paronychium): The skin that folds over the nail on three sides around it

- Nail Plate: The visible, tough outer surface of the nail

Terms and Conditions

Our fingernails are an indicator of many medical conditions. Awareness of changes in color, shape, and texture of the nail can lead to early detection of multiple diseases:

Argyria: a condition resulting after a person ingests the element silver (Ag) and causes the nails to become a blue-gray color

Beau's Lines: horizontal depressions in the nail which indicate periods of decreased growth in the nailbed. Seen in people with eczema, among other conditions

Blue Nails: may indicate heart disease

Brittle Nails: signify possible iron deficiency and thyroid problems, impaired renal functions, and circulatory disorders

Broad Nails: may indicate problems with hormone balance

Clubbing of the fingers: bulbous enlargement of the distal portion of the fingers; early sign of an underlying disease

<u>Dark and Thin Nails</u>: may indicate a vitamin B12 deficiency

<u>Half and Half Nails</u>: a partially pink and white nail may indicate kidney disease

<u>Koilonychia</u>: deformity in the nail causing concavity and a spoon like appearance. A known clinical symptom of iron deficiency

<u>Leukonychia</u>: white spots on the nailplate

<u>Muehrcke's Nails</u>: chronic hypoalbuminemia

<u>Onychia</u>: inflammation of the nail matrix

<u>Onycholysis</u>: the separation or loosening of a fingernail from its nail bed, most often starting at the tip of the nail

<u>Onychomycosis (tinea unguium)</u>: fungal infection of the nail caused by yeast, dermaphytes, and nondermaphytes. Causes the nail to become thick and often an opaque color

<u>Paronychia</u>: infection at the nail fold and the skin around the nail. Can be caused by trauma to that area, fungus, or yeast

<u>Phototoxic Nails</u>: result from the combination of extensive exposure to sunlight in conjunction with certain oral medications

<u>Pliant Nails</u>: may indicate rheumatoid arthritis

<u>Psoriasiform changes</u>: nail pitting

<u>Ridges/Grooves</u>: may indicated a renal disorder or iron deficiency

<u>Subungual hematoma</u>: a direct injury to the nail causes blood to accumulate under the nail

<u>Terry's Nails</u>: white nails with the absence of the lunula, found in people with alcoholic cirrhosis

<u>White Nails</u>: may indicate a liver disease

<u>Yellow Nails</u>: may indicate internal disorders long before other symptoms appears, including disorders of the lymphatic system, respiratory

disorders, diabetes, and liver disorders; yellow nails are often noted in the tobacco abuse

Interesting facts about fingernails

- Fingernails grow faster in the summer than in the winter

- Nails grow an average of 0.1 mm each day

- Fingernails grow faster than toenails

FINGERPRINTING

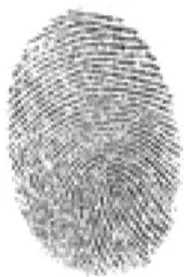

The use of fingerprints has been traced as far back as 14th century Persia, where it was used on government officials, and continues to play an important role for today's law enforcement.

The scientific study of papillary ridges of the hands and feet is credited as beginning with the work of Joannes Evangelista Purkinje, a Czech physiologist and biologist in 1823. In 1892 Sir Francis Galton published his classic treaties on fingerprints.

Conventionally, a fingerprint is formed by coating the "friction ridges," the raised parts of the epidermis, with ink and rubbing the finger along a smooth surface like paper. Fingerprint identification compares the fingerprints in question to known fingerprints using biometric technology, though the process is complicated by the fact that no two fingerprints ever look the same.

With new analytical technology, utilizing mass spectrometry, a fingerprint can now reveal more than the identity of a person. It can also identify what the person has been touching, including drugs, explosive, or poisons.

To standardize the fingerprinting process, **fingers are numbered from 1 to 10, with the right thumb as number 1 and the left thumb as number 6.**

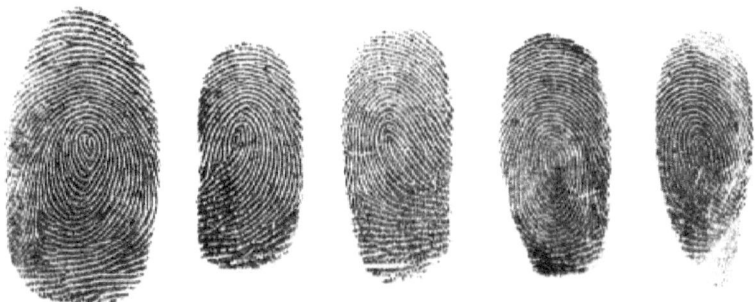

On the official applicant form produced by the Federal Bureau of Investigation of the U.S. Department of Justice, the instructions to obtain "classifiable" fingerprints are as follows:

Directions for the applicant:
1. use black printer's ink
2. distribute ink evenly on inking slab
3. wash and dry fingers thoroughly
4. roll fingers from nail to nail
5. be sure impressions are recorded in correct order
6. if an amputation or a deformity makes it impossible to print a finger, make a notation to that effect in the individual finger block
7. if some physical condition makes it impossible to obtain perfect impressions, submit the best that can be obtained with a memo stapled to the card explaining the circumstances
8. examine the completed prints to see if they can be classified, bearing in mind that most fingerprints fall into the patterns shown on this card

GLOVES

A glove is an article of clothing worn on the hand characterized by separate openings for the fingers.

Gloves with openings for the fingers but no covering are called "fingerless gloves," while those which cover the fingers but do not have separate openings are called "mittens." Fingerless gloves without separate openings are known as "gauntlets."

SPORTS GLOVES

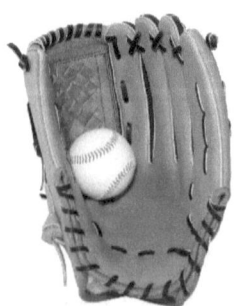

- **baseball glove**: The baseball glove, or mitt, has gone through several important transformations since its first documented use in 1875 by Charles Waitt, an outfielder and first baseman for the St. Louis Cardinals. Though the first players to use a mitt were taunted as being "too soft," the glove was slowly accepted but gradually developed into the essential piece of equipment it is today. The first gloves, made of scraps of leather sewn together over a player's hand, were designed to knock down, rather than catch, the baseball. Later models added padding, seams to separate the fingers, and other details that improved both safety and comfort. Eventually, variations of the glove were developed for the different positions, including first base, outfield, infield, pitcher and catcher.

Towards the end of the 1870s, several players started using gloves with added protection, which were useful for their specific positions. In the 1880s, the catcher's "puff pillow" glove first appeared, complete with a layer of leather to cover the wool padding. In 1883, Canadian-American shortstop Arthur Irwin popularized the mitt with his creation of the infielders' glove. The shape and size of the glove continued to evolve over the years, and in 1990, Major League Baseball enforced limits on the length of gloves by position for the first time.

Though the glove has not changed much in the modern era, thanks to today's baseball technology (and corporate sponsorship), professional baseball players have the ability to "customize" their glove to provide the perfect fit. Veteran relief pitcher Armando Benitez, for example, uses a specially designed glove that allows him to keep two fingers through an extra-large "fingerhood" located in the back.

- **boxing gloves**: Boxing gloves are used to cushion impact during boxing matches. Offensively, they protect the knuckles of the fighters, while defensively; they are used to block punches from an opponent, primarily to the head. Though ancient versions of the boxing glove were used by the Greeks and Romans over three thousand years ago, boxing gloves were officially introduced to professional fights as an adaptation to boxing rules in 1867. The gloves were adopted as a safety improvement to bare-knuckle fights, though these fights continued after the gloves' inception. Types of boxing gloves include the *speed glove*, the *bag glove*, the *sparring glove* and the *fight glove*. Speed gloves are light mittens designed to protect fighters from scrapes and bruises while hitting a speed bag or other lightweight bag. Bag gloves contain extra cushioning for use with punching bags and other heavier bags. Sparring and fight gloves are worn during practice and professional fights, respectively, and are weighted to reduce swing speed for safety purposes.

- **golf glove**: Golf gloves are used to add grip and prevent blisters. Players traditionally wear one glove on their opposite hand (e.g. on the left hand for a right-handed person).

- **hockey gloves**: Though it is unclear who introduced the hockey glove to the game, its rationale is obvious: warmth and protection. By 1900, players began to add extra padding to the glove. The goalie glove remained the same as that of the other players until 1915, when special padding was added. Between 1925 and 1930, a goalie glove with a hard outer cage was created, called "the Blocker." A different goalie glove, "the Catcher," was added in 1948, so named because its creator, Chicago Blackhawks goalie Ernie Francis, attached a first baseman's mitt to the back of his hockey glove, and other goalies soon followed. To determine your hockey glove size, measure between your fingertips to your elbow.

MEDICAL GLOVES

- **medical gloves**: Medical gloves' primary purpose is safety. The two main types of gloves are exam and surgical, the latter being made to higher specifications, including size. The gloves aim to ensure sanitary conditions and limit the spread of disease through interpersonal contact. They are usually made of latex and lubricated with powdered cornstarch, though non-powdered gloves are not being used during surgery to prevent any potential interference to the healing process caused by the cornstarch. For those allergic to latex, non-latex gloves made of vinyl or other material are often utilized.

WORK GLOVES

- Gloves used for doing heavy duty work in construction zones, car mechanic work, and lawn and garden labor is vital to avoid injuries. A study by the Liberty Mutual Research Institute for

Safety shows that wearing gloves reduced the risk of injury to the hand by sixty percent. The Occupational Safety and Health Administration (OSHA) advises that with appropriate gloves, finger injuries can be avoided.

KINESIOLOGY

Finger motions include extension, flexion, abduction, adduction, and circumduction; thumb motion also includes opposition.

MOTION TERMINOLOGY[12]

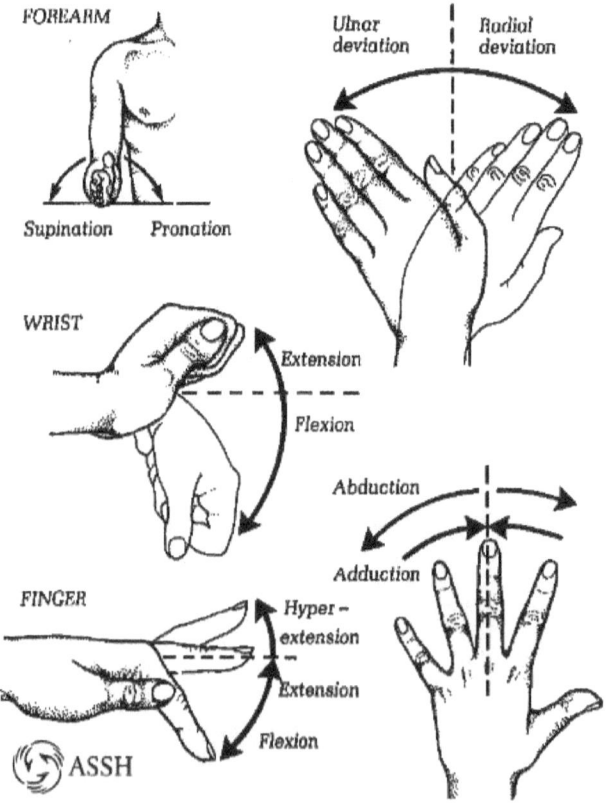

12 Images © 2002 American Society for Surgery of the Hand *Essentials of Hand Surgery*

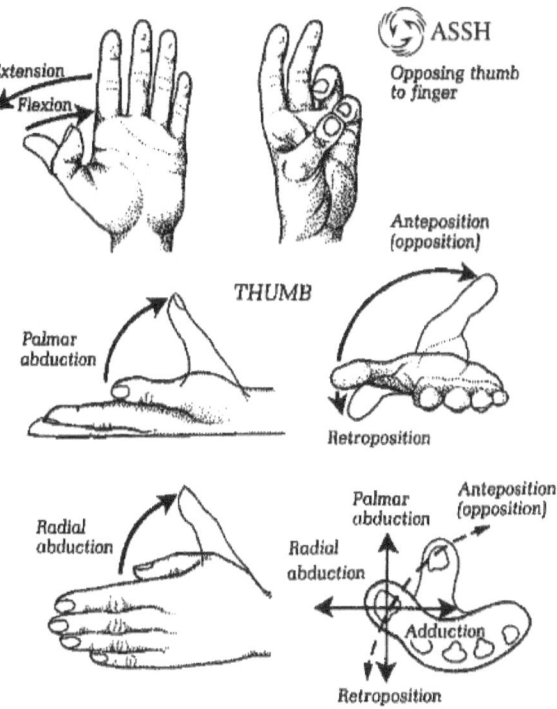

ASSH

Articulationes Digitorum Manus; Interphalangeal Joints)[13]

The interphalangeal articulations are hinge-joints; each has a volar and two collateral ligaments. The arrangement of these ligaments is similar to those in the metacarpophalangeal articulations. The Extensor tendons supply the place of posterior ligaments.

Movements.—The only movements permitted in the interphalangeal joints are flexion and extension; these movements are more extensive between the first and second phalanges than between the second and third. The amount of flexion is very considerable, but extension is limited by the volar and collateral ligaments.

Muscles Acting on the Joints of the Digits.—Flexion of the metacarpophalangeal joints of the fingers is effected by the Flexor digitorum sublimis and profundus, Lumbricales, and Interossei, assisted in the case of the little finger by the Flexor digiti quinti brevis.

13 Henry Gray, Anatomy of the Human Body, 1918. With permission of Bartleby.com

Extension is produced by the Extensor digitorum communis, Extensor indicis proprius, and Extensor digiti quinti proprius.

Flexion of the interphalangeal joints of the fingers is accomplished by the Flexor digitorum profundus acting on the proximal and distal joints and by the Flexor digitorum sublimis acting on the proximal joints. Extension is effected mainly by the Lumbricales and Interossei, the long Extensors having little or no action upon these joints.

Flexion of the metacarpophalangeal joint of the thumb is effected by the Flexor pollicis longus and brevis; extension by the Extensor pollicis longus and brevis. Flexion of the interphalangeal joint is accomplished by the Flexor pollicis longus, and extension by the Extensor pollicis longus.

LANGUAGES

The **Anglo- Saxons** had specific names for the fingers:

-   thumb: thuma
-   index finger: towcher (meaning the finger that touches)
-   middle finger: long man
-   ring finger: gold finger
-   little finger: ear finger

Armenian

-   thumb: butmat
-   index finger: tsutsamat
-   middle finger: megnamat
-   ring finger: matnemat
-   little finger: chaqueet

Azarbaijani

-   thumb: bash
-   pointer finger: shahadat barmag
-   middle finger: orta barmag
-   ring finger: adsiz barmag
-   little finger: chochala barmag

Bulgarian

- thumb: palez
- index finger: pokazaletz
- middle finger: freden palez
- ring finger: bezeimenen
- little finger: meizetinetz

Catalan

- thumb: polze
- index finger: index
- middle finger: cor
- ring finger: anular
- little finger: menovell

Comorian

- finger: shaya
- fingers: zaya
- thumb: shaya shakaowo

Croatian

- thumb: palac
- index finger: kaziprst
- middle finger: srednji prst
- ring finger: prstenjak
- little finger: mali prst

Czech

- thumb: palec
- index finger: ukazovák
- middle finger: prostředník
- ring finger: prsteník
- little finger: malíček

Dutch

- thumb: Dium
- index finger: wijsvinger
- middle finger: middlevinger
- ring finger: ringvinger
- little finger: pink

Farsi

- thumb: angushteh bowzowrg
- index finger: angushteh neshaneh
- middle finger: angushteh vasat
- ring finger: angushteh chaharum
- little finger: angushteh qucheck

Finnish

- thumb: peukalo
- index finger: esusormi
- middle finger: keskisormi
- ring finger: nimeton
- little finger: pikkusormi

French

- thumb: Le pouce
- index finger: L'index
- middle finger: L'medius
- ring finger: L'annulaire
- little finger: L'auriculaire
- finger: doigt

German

- thumb: daumen
- index finger: zeigefinger
- middle finger: mittelfinger
- ring finger: ringfinger
- little finger: kleinfinger
- digit: ziffer

Hebrew

- thumb: agudal
- index finger: etsba mora
- middle finger: ama
- ring finger: qmitsa
- little finger:zeret
- finger: etsba

Hungarian

- thumb: nagy ujj
- index finger: mutató ujj
- middle finger: középső ujj
- ring finger: gyűrűs ujj
- little finger: kis ujj

Indonesian

- thumb: jempol
- index finger: telunjuk
- middle finger: jari tengah
- ring finger: jari cincin
- little finger: kelingking
- finger: jari

Irish

- thumb: ordog
- index finger: corrmhear
- middle finger: mear fhada
- ring finger: mear fainne
- little finger: luidin

Italian

- thumb: pollice
- index finger: dito indice
- middle finger: dito medio
- ring finger: anulare
- little finger: dito piccolo
- finger: dito

Japanese

- thumb: oya-yubi
- index finger: hitosashi-yubi
- middle finger: naka-yubi
- ring finger: kusri-yubi
- little finger: ko-yubi

** For medical purposes, the Japanese use the term digits when referring to fingers:

- first digit: dai-ichi-shi
- second digit: dai-ni-shi
- third digit: dai-san-shi

Latin

- thumb: Polex
- index finger: demonstratus
- middle finger: impudicus
- ring finger: annularis
- little finger: auricularis

Latvian

- thumb: Ikskis
- index finger: Raditajpirksts
- middle finger: Videjais Pirksts
- ring finger: Zeltnesis
- little finger: Mazais Pirksts

Malay

- thumb: Ibu jari
- index finger: Jari Telunjuk
- middle finger: Jari Hantu
- ring finger: Jari Manis
- little finger: Jari Kelingking

Portuguese

- thumb: polegar
- index finger: indicador
- middle finger: do meio
- ring finger: anular
- little finger:minimo

Romanian

- thumb: degetul mare
- index finger: aratatorul
- middle finger: degetul mijlociu
- ring finger: inelarul
- little finger: degetul mic

Slovenian

- thumb: palec
- index finger: kazalec
- middle finger: sredinec
- ring finger: prstanec
- little finger: mezinec

Spanish

- thumb: pulgar
- index finger: dedo indice
- middle finger: dedo medio
- ring finger: dedo anular
- little finger: dedo pequeno
- finger: dedo

Swedish

- thumb: tumme
- index finger: pekfinger
- middle finger: langfinger
- ring finger: ringfinger
- little finger:litten finger

Turkish

- thumb: basparmak
- index finger: indeksini yapmak

Welsh

- thumb:bawd
- index finger: bys tored
- middle finger: bys canol
- ring finger: bys y fodrwy
- little finger: bys bach

MEDICAL CODING

The Current Procedural Coding (CPT) book published on an annual basis by the American Medical Association (AMA) is used by physicians to identify the procedures and services provided by them to the patient. It is copyrighted by the AMA.

The foreword of the CPT states, "it is a listing of descriptive terms and identifying codes for reporting medical services and procedures performed by physicians. The purpose of the terminology is to provide a uniform language that will accurately describe medical, surgical, and diagnostic services, and will thereby provide an effective means for reliable nationwide communication among physicians, patients, and third parties."

ICD-9-CM is the abbreviation for International Classification of Diseases, 9th edition, and Clinical Modification. It is a reference for reporting diagnostic codes.

CPT codes consist of five-digit numbers which represent individual services and procedures. These codes may be further defined by modifiers to help explain an unusual circumstance or specificity associated with a service or procedure.

The following modifiers are required when reporting services performed on the digits of the hands:

Anatomical Site	*Description by CPT code book*	
Thumb, left hand		**FA**
Index finger, left hand	Left hand, second digit	**F1**
Long finger, left hand	Left hand, third digit	**F2**
Ring finger, left hand	Left hand, fourth digit	**F3**
Little finger, left hand	Left hand fifth digit	**F4**
Thumb, right hand		**F5**
Index finger, right hand	Right hand, second digit	**F6**
Long finger, right hand	Right hand, third digit	**F7**
Ring finger, right hand	Right hand, fourth digit	**F8**
Little finger, right hand	Right hand, fifth digit	**F9**

Music

Musicians do not use the same nomenclature for naming the fingers as surgeons. Even amongst themselves, their methodology varies by instrument.

There are various methods of **fingering** used across all areas of music. The fingering technique is used to denote the correct finger placement on a particular instrument:

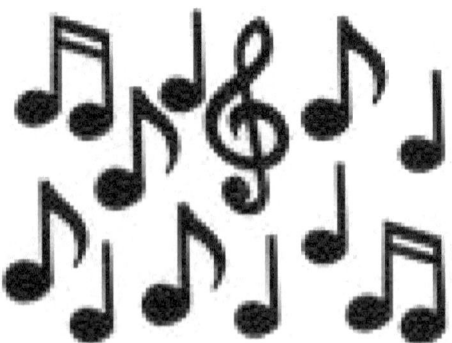

Drums

When holding drum sticks, there are two main grips that drummers use. First is the conventional grip, where the dominant hand holds the stick near the bottom with the thumb and index fingers, the other fingers simply rest on the stick. With the non-dominant hand, the index and middle fingers are placed on the top of the stick, the other two fingers are placed under the stick, and the thumb is placed on the index finger. Second is the matched grip, where both hands are held in the same position as the right hand is in the conventional grip.

Guitar

In learning the guitar, the initial training is usually with strumming the chords. Then coming up with an effective fretting-hand fingering plan is an essential part of guitar playing.

Typically, the fretting hand index finger is referred to as the *first* *finger*; the middle finger is called the *second finger*; the ring finger is known as the *third finger*; and the little finger or "pinky" is called the *fourth finger*.

For finger identification the left hand is numbered 1 to 4 with the index finger being number 1 and the little finger being number 4. The right hand fingers are denoted by the first letter of the Spanish word for each finger: pulgar (thumb), indicio (index), medio (middle), and anular (ring).

Piano

Numbers are commonly used to teach beginning pianists proper placement of their fingers on the piano keys.

Pianists label the fingers 1 through 5, including the thumb as finger number 1.

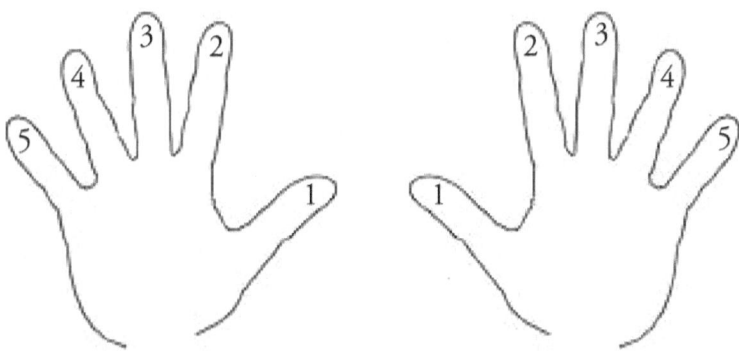

For more advanced pianists, fingering plays an important role in the proper execution of a piece. "The Virtuoso Pianist in 60 Exercises" by 19th-century composer Charles-Louis Hanon, a compilation of short exercises meant to train pianists in fingering and flexibility, remains a critical component of any serious player's practice regimen. Though pianists often form their own opinion concerning fingering for any given piece, there are often areas in more difficult pieces that require a specific technique in order to be played. In addition, Bach and other classical composers did not dictate proper fingering technique for their pieces, leaving that task to musical editors and piano students of future generations. Thus, fingering is central to the performance of pieces on the piano.

Violin

With violin players, the fingers are called: thumb, with the index finger designated as the 1st finger; the middle finger as the 2nd finger; the ring finger as the 3rd finger; and the little finger as the 4th finger.

For instance, according to Professor Emery Erdlee's book, Mastery of the Bow, he states that there are numerous techniques to hold the bow when playing the violin:

- Franco-Belgian School: "the index finger should come into contact with the stick at the extreme end of the joint,…space between index and middle fingers, thumb opposite middle finger, bow hair at excessive tension"

- German School: "put the first joint of the first finger in contact with the wood"

- Russian School: " put the tick at the top of the third joint of the first finger, nearly into the palm with the hand naturally tilted"

Professor Erdlee writes, "To test and develop strength of the individual fingers, practice long tones, holding the bow between the thumb and various finger combinations, while other fingers are suspended above the stick.

Thumb and 1st and 2nd fingers.
Thumb and 2nd and 3rd fingers
Thumb and 3rd and 4th fingers…."

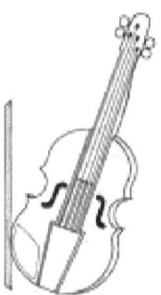

Nursery Rhymes

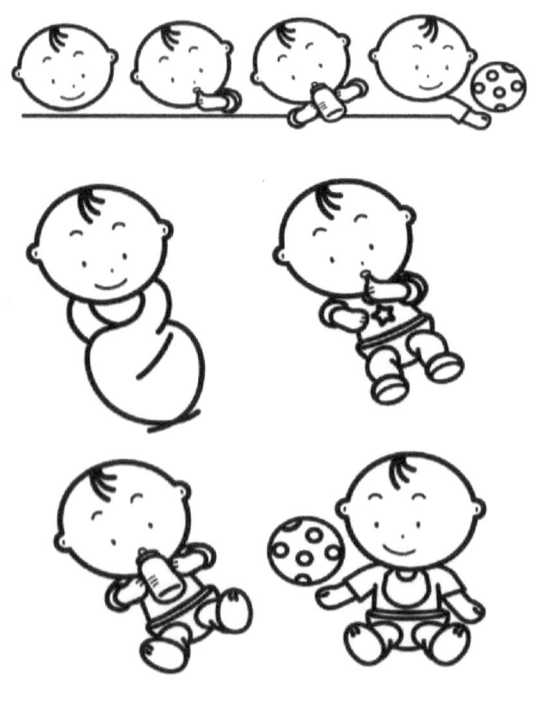

From an early age, children are exposed to various ditties that are composed for easy recognition of the fingers. Finger rhymes and finger plays are used with preschool-aged children to help associate fingers with names, which enhances their recall abilities. These rhymes and rotes are associated with finger plays for enhancement with visual effects

Ironically, children learn various names for the fingers at different stages of development, which may help explain some of the confusion as adults.

Tommy Thumb

One great example is "Tommy Thumb," a nursery rhyme that utilizes mnemonic devices in order to teach children the names of the fingers. Each finger takes on a different persona:

The thumb - Tommy Thumb

The index finger - Peter Pointer

The middle finger - Toby Tall

The ring finger -Ruby Ring

The small finger -Baby Small

Tommy thumb, Tommy thumb,
Where are you?
Here I am, Here I am,
How are you?

Repeat with all the fingers: ***POINTER, TALL MAN, RING MAN,***
OR SMALLMAN or PINKIE

Peter pointer, Peter pointer,
Where are you?
Here I am, Here I am,
How are you?

Toby tall, Toby tall,
Where are you?
Here I am, Here I am,
How are you?

Ruby ring, Ruby ring,
Where are you?
Here I am, Here I am,
How are you?

Baby small, Baby small,
Where are you?
Here I am, Here I am,
How are you?

Fingers all, Fingers all,
Where are you?
Here I am, Here I am,
How are you?

Another example of a "finger" nursery rhyme is:

Where is Thumbkin

Where is thumbkin?
Where is thumbkin?
Here I am!
Here I am!
How are you today, sir?
Very well, I thank you.
Run away.
Run away.

(Repeat with each finger: pointer, tall man, ringman, and pinky.)

Ten Fingers

I have ten fingers   (hold up both hands, fingers spread)
And they all belong to me, (point to self)
I can make them do things-
Would you like to see?

I can shut them up tight   (make fists)
I can open them wide   (open hands)
I can put them together   (place palms together)

I can make them all hide   (put hands behind back)

I can make them jump high   (hands over head)
I can make them jump low   (touch floor)
I can fold them up quietly   (fold hands in lap)
And hold them just so.

This Old Man

This old man, he played one.
He played knick-knack on his thumb.
With a knick-knack paddy whack,
Give your dog a bone.
This old man came rolling home.

Five Little Birdies

Five little birdies, flying around our door,

(five fingers one hand up in the air, as verse is said other hand bends down each finger)

The blue one flew away and then there were four.

Four little birdies sitting in a tree,
The yellow one flew away and then there were three.

The little birdies didn't know what to do,
So the red one flew away, and then there were two.

Two little birdies sitting in the sun,
The Brown one flew away, and there was one.

The little green birdie felt so all alone,
He/she flew away and then there was none.

Later on that very day,
five little birdies came back to play.

Hillary J. Kener and Dr. Michael Zeide

Five Fat Peas

Five fat peas in a pea pod pressed
(children hold hand in a fist)

One grew, two grew, so did all the rest.
(put thumb and fingers up one by one)
They grew and grew
(raise hand in the air very slowly)

And did not stop,
Until one day
The pod went POP!
(children clap hands together)

Five Little Monkeys

Five little monkeys jumping
on the bed
One fell off and bumped
his head
Mama called the doctor and
the doctor Said,
"No more monkeys
jumping on the bed!
Four little monkeys jumping
on the bed, three little monkeys jumping on the bed, (and so on).

PALMISTRY

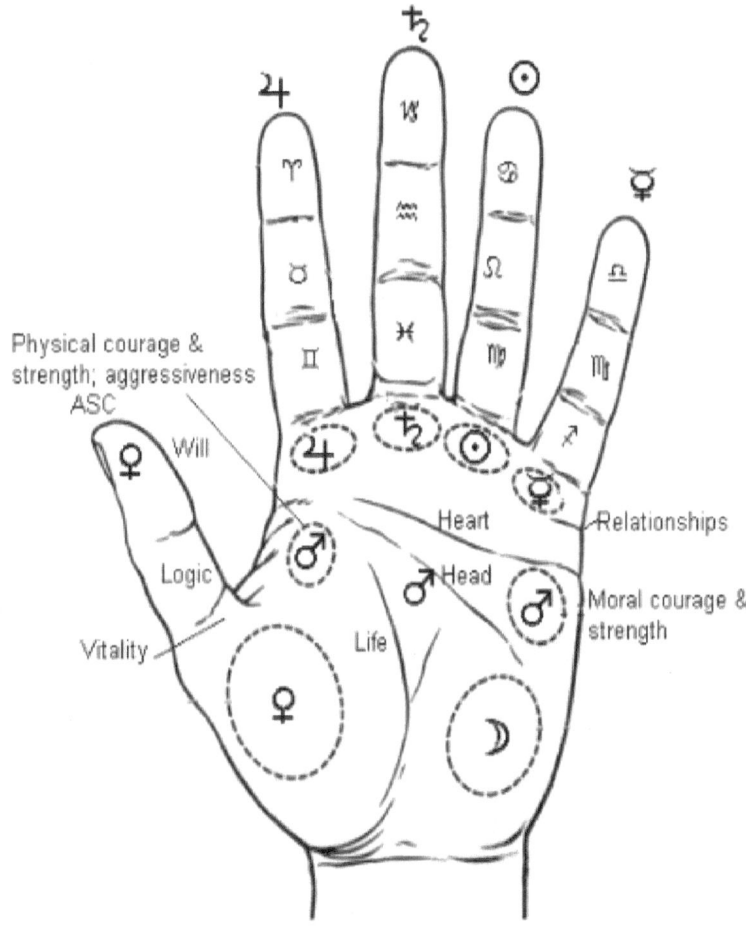

14 Courtesy of Anne Massey

The origin of palmistry can date back to about 5000 years ago, when it was practiced by Hindu astrologers. Palmistry later spread to China and Egypt, and then Europe in the 12ᵗʰ century.

This ancient practice uses the hand as a source of knowledge, revealing one's future and personal characteristics. As part of the palm-reading process, each of the fingers is associated with Greek gods and goddesses and therefore given unique qualities pertaining to the person.

Palm-reading is also known as palmistry, hand analysis and cheiromancy, the latter coming from the Greek words *cheir*, meaning hand, and *manteia*, meaning divination. According to the ancient practice, by charting the astrological correspondences found in the hands and understanding the mythologies of the gods and planets associated with each part of that map, it is possible to understand yourself and others by making simple observations about thumb size, finger length, gesture, lines and skin color.

The *astrological map* of the hand is the key to palm reading.[15] Without an understanding of the qualities that correspond to each part of the hand and each finger, the lines, dots, squares, cuts, hollows and bumps are meaningless. A star on the mound of Apollo has a very different meaning from a star on the mound of Mars. A person with a large thumb and a long, straight Jupiter finger will behave very differently than a person with a large thumb and a short, twisted Jupiter.

The astrological map of the hand is the basis upon which the highways and byways of the nervous system become etched. A firm grasp of the meanings and myths associated with each area is the basis for the study of palmistry.

The *mounds* and *fingers* were named for the seven planets that were recognized by astronomers and astrologers at an earlier time in our history. Some modern palmists have added the outer planets, Uranus, Neptune and Pluto, to the map.

---

15 Courtesy of Leslie Zemenek

The following are terms used in the palm-reading process related specifically to fingers:

Astrological Finger Names:

Jupiter: The index finger and the mound below it
Saturn: The middle finger and the mound below it
Apollo: The ring finger and the mound below it
Mercury: The little finger and the mound below it

Explanation for the astrological finger names:

The fingers are named for the mythological figures who display qualities of the specific finger.

- <u>Jupiter</u>: the index finger is named after the leader of the world, Jupiter. It is associated with ambition and drive.
- <u>Saturn</u>: the middle finger is named after the father of Jupiter, Saturn. He represents knowledge, as does this finger.
- <u>Apollo</u>: the ring finger is named after the sun god, Apollo. It is associated with talent.
- <u>Mercury</u>: the little finger is named after the messenger of the gods, Mercury. This finger is associated with communication.

Definitions of miscellaneous palmistry terms:

- Chirognomy- the study of hand shapes, including the size and shapes of the fingers and mounds

- Cheiromancy- the study of the lines in the hands. This word is also often used to describe the entire study of palmistry.

- Dermatoglyphics- scientific study of finger ridges

- Interdigital area- region between two fingers

- Phalange- the finger

- Radial- radial side of the palm is the thumb side

- Solomon's Ring- a line circulating the index finger

- Ulna- the ulnar side of the palm is the little finger side

Explanation of Finger Lengths in Palmistry

In palm reading, different characteristics are assigned to finger lengths:

Jupiter, Index Finger:

-A long index finger indicates a person who shows poise and self-belief. These individuals often feel extremely self-secure and like to have the dominant position.

-A short index finger indicates an introverted and non-confident person.

-An arced index finger indicates a person has many pastime activities and enjoys accumulating goods.

Saturn, Middle Finger:

-A long middle finger signifies an extremely determined person.

-A short middle finger signifies a more carefree individual with not much drive.

-A middle finger that is an intermediate size signifies a good balance between both personality extremes.

Apollo, Ring Finger:

-A long ring finger designates a person with an artsy edge.

-A short ring finger is not seen very often.

Mercury, Little Finger:

-A long little finger represents an intelligent person. Many of these people are very articulate and make fine authors.

-A short little finger represents child-like responses to situations.

-A little finger located low on the hand represents a person who has had struggles with his or her parents.

-A little finger protruding from the hand represents a person stuck in a loveless courtship.

SIGN LANGUAGE

Just as the eyes are the window to the soul, for the deaf community, the fingers are a window to communication. Used by millions, sign language is a visual, "living language." Though the language varies worldwide, an individual sign is always comprised of three basic components: the sign, the motion of the hands, and the position of the body.

Indian Sign Language

Since Native American Indians often spoke many different languages, they frequently used sign language to communicate. Each hand or finger gesture had a different significance and this form of communication was primarily used by the Plains Indians which is why it is sometimes known as "Plains sign talk."

American Sign Language

The following is a textual description of the official American Sign Language (ASL) alphabet.

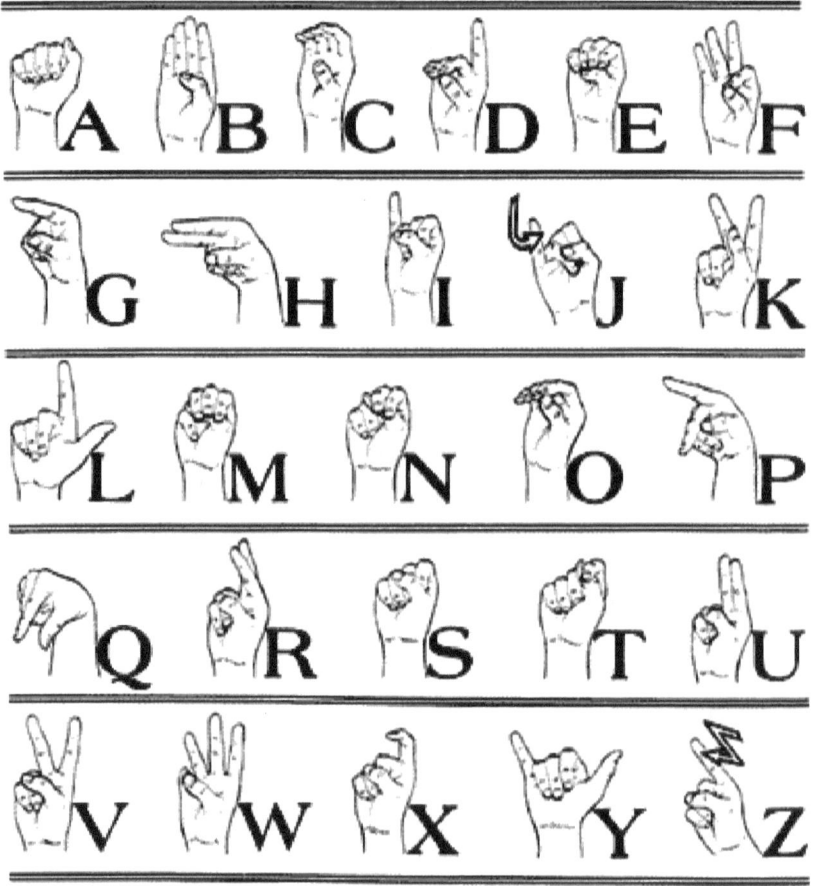

- **A**: A closed fist, all finger folded against the palm, thumb is straight, alongside the index finger.
- **B**: All fingers are straight. Thumb is folded across palm.
- **C**: All fingers partially folded. Thumb is partially folded. Hand is turn slightly to the left so viewer can see backward "C" shape formed by thumb and index finger.
- **D**: Middle, ring and little fingers are partially folded. Tip of thumb is touching tip of middle finger. Index finger is straight. Hand is turned slightly so viewer can see "d" shape formed by thumb, middle and index fingers.
- **E**: Thumb is folded across in front of palm but not touching it. All fingers are partially folded with the tips of index, middle

and ring fingers touching the thumb between the knuckle and the tip.

- **F**: Tip of index finger is touching tip of thumb. Middle, ring and little fingers are straight and slightly spread.

- **G**: Middle, ring and little fingers are folded down across palm. Thumb is straight but pulled in so that it is in front of the index finger. The index finger is straight and pointing forwards slightly so that it is parallel to the thumb, The thumb and index finger are not touching. The whole hand is turned towards the left and tilted slightly so the thumb and index finger are towards the viewer and pointing up at about 45 degrees.

- **H**: Ring and little finger are folded down. Thumb is folded over ring and little finger. Index finger and middle finger are straight and together. The hand is tilted over so that the fingers are horizontal and pointing to the left.

- **I**: Index, middle and ring fingers are folded down. Thumb is folded across index middle and ring fingers. Little finger is straight.

- **J**: Index, middle and ring fingers are folded down. Thumb is folded across index middle and ring fingers. Little finger is straight. The hand is moved so that little finger draws a "J" shape. Motion is a curve moving forward and then right. The hand turns to the right.

- **K**: Ring and little fingers are folded down. Index and middle finger are straight and slightly spread. Thumb is straight and pointing up to the middle finger. (This is very similar to V the only difference is the position of the thumb.

- **L**: Middle, ring and little finger are folded down over palm. Index finger and thumb are straight. Thumb is sticking out sideways at 90 degrees to index finger to form "L" shape.

- **M**: Little finger is folded. Thumb is folded across to touch little finger. Index, middle and ring fingers are folded down over thumb.

- **N**: Little and ring finger are folded. Thumb is folded across ring and little finger. Index finger and middle finger are folded down over thumb.

- **O**: All fingers are partially folded. Thumb is partially folded and tip of thumb is touching tip of index finger. Hand is turned slightly so viewer can see "O" shape formed by thumb and index finger.

- **P**: Ring and little finger are folded down. Index finger is straight. Middle finger is straight but pointing forward so that is at 90 degrees to index finger. Tip of thumb is touching middle of middle finger. Hand is turned to the left and twisted over so that index finger is horizontal and middle finger is pointing down. Viewer can (sort of) see a "P" shape formed by middle finger and thumb.

- **Q**: Ring and little fingers are folded down across palm. Thumb is straight but pulled in so that it is in front of the index finger. The index finger is straight and pointing forwards slightly so that it is parallel to the thumb. The index finger and thumb are not touching. The Middle finger is bent down and across to the right of the thumb. The whole hand is turned towards the left and tilted so the thumb and index finger are towards the viewer and pointing almost straight down.

- **R**: Ring and little finger are folded against the palm, held down by thumb, index and middle finger are straight and crossed, index finger in front.

- **S**: Clenched fist. All fingers folded tightly into palm. Thumb is across index and middle fingers.

- **T**: Middle, ring and little fingers are fold down across palm. Thumb is folded across middle finger. Index finger is folded over thumb.

- **U**: Ring and little finger are folded against the palm, held down by thumb, index and middle finger are straight and together.

- **V**: Ring and little finger fold against the palm, held down by thumb, index and middle finger are straight and spread to form a "V" shape.

- **W**: Tip of little finger is touching tip of thumb. Index, middle and ring fingers are straight and slightly spread.

- **X:** Middle, ring and little fingers are folded down. Index finger is bent at both joints. Thumb is pulled in and slightly bent at the joint. The hand is turned to the left so view can see thumb and index finger.

- **Y**: Index, middle and ring ringers folded against palm. Little finger and thumb are straight and spread wide.

- **Z**: Middle, ring and little fingers are folded. Thumb is folded across middle and ring fingers. Index finger is straight. The hand is moved so that the tip of index finger draws out a "Z" shape. The motion is (1) from right to left. (2) from left to right and forward. (3) from right to left.

SPORTS

With the notable exception of soccer, we rely heavily on our fingers in the majority of sports. From baseball to basketball, and swimming to softball, the positioning of our fingers plays an important role in playing correctly and avoiding injury. In many sports, the way we grip equipment can be the difference between mediocre play and maximal performance.

Baseball: The basic throwing grip used by all positions, including the pitcher, is the four-seam grip, named so because all four seams spin consecutively. To throw a four-seam fastball, place your middle and index fingers across the "horseshoe seam" of the baseball, with the fingertips resting atop the seam and the horseshoe facing inward (e.g. to the left for a right-handed thrower). Your thumb should be placed directly under the baseball, while your ring and little fingers rest to the side. Held somewhat loosely and with the proper grip, the four-seam fastball should maximize velocity and accuracy.

Pitchers, whose aim is to confuse and confound the batter, have developed other grips than allow for variance in both velocity and straightness, most notably the two-seam fastball, change-up, curveball, knuckleball, knuckle curveball, slider, split-finger, and palm ball.

Basketball: In addition to balance and leg positioning, hand and finger position is an important component of properly shooting the basketball. For the "set shot" position, the ball should be held with your dominant hand under the ball and other hand on the side of the ball, the former propelling the basketball towards to the basket and the latter giving it direction. Your fingers should be spread out evenly, and your elbow should be held beneath the basketball, creating a catapult-like shooting motion.

Golf: There are three main grips in golf: the overlap grip, the interlock grip, and the 10-finger grip.

- *the overlap*: most golfers use this type of grip. Correct positioning involves the little finger of the right hand resting on the index finger of the left hand.
- *the interlock*: the fingers overlap; best suited for golfers with large hands
- *the 10 finger grip:* best suited for golfers with small hands, also known as the baseball grip

Horseback Riding: The two main ways to hold the reins are the Western grip and the English grip:

- *Western*: Hold the reins in one hand with the thumb atop the index finger's knuckle.
- *English*: Hold each rein with the little and ring finger, with thumb pointed up

Marbles: In the world of professional marbles games, nothing is more sacred than a player's thumb and index finger, as the grip is inviolable.

Softball: Like in baseball, softball players generally use a four-seam grip (see "Baseball" above) and pitchers vary this grip to allow for changes in speed and direction. Two of the variations:

- *Drop ball*: Take thumb off of ball right before releasing it and snap wrist over ball. A downward spin is initiated when the fingers roll over the ball.
- *Knuckleball*: tuck the middle three fingers under, the thumb and little finger let go of the ball upon release and the three knuckles push the ball out.

Swimming: In freestyle swimming, the general rule of thumb is that the fingers be held together as you swim, like a paddle propelling you through the water. This technique minimizes surface area, thus minimizing water resistance, though some say the fingers should be slightly separated in order to create a more relaxed hand position.

Tennis: The tennis grip varies for beginners and experts as it does for forehand and backhand shots. The most common grips:

1. *Eastern forehand grip* – Also known as the "Handshake grip," this grip may be used for any shot but is most popularly used for serves and volleys. To form this grip, hold the handle of the racket with your dominant hand as if shaking someone's hand, with the strings of the racket perpendicular to the ground. This should create a "V" formation between your index and thumb, with the other fingers gripping the racket from underneath and the big knuckle of your index finger lying atop the racket.

2. *Continental grip* – A variation of the Eastern forehand grip used by more advanced players, this grip is formed by using the same hand position but slightly tilting the racket to about the "11 o'clock" position (1 o'clock for a left-handed player). This allows for more variations in spin.

3. *Western forehand grip* – Similar to the Continental grip, this grip is produced with the "V-formation" slightly tilted inward for both forehand and backhand shots to varying degrees.

4. *Two-handed grips* – These grips generally rely on the standard "V-shaped" grip of the dominant hand joined by a second hand held in varying positions.

String Figure Nomenclature

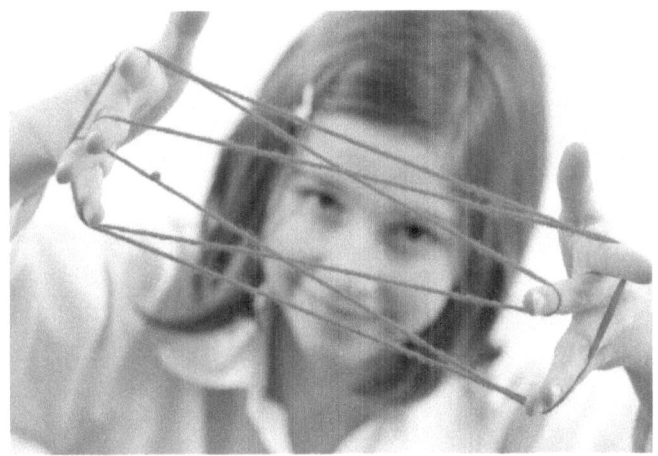

Making string figures is an art involving the intricate looping, bending, and extension of strings of various lengths. String figures have a specific nomenclature.

Naming of the hands and fingers:

L- left
R-right
H-hand

1-thumb
2-index
3-middle

4-ring
5-little

The hand letter is written first, followed by the finger number.
    Example: L2 is left index

Naming of the strings and loops:

u before finger name- upper
l before finger name-lower

n following finger name- near
f following finger name- far

Naming of Actions:

Caroline extension- raise string with finger 2 and grab it with finger 1; used when there is a loop on finger 1

Hook down- obtain the string using the palm side of the finger

Hook up- obtain the string using the palm side of the finger and rotating the finger   halfway in either direction

Pick up- obtain the string using the dorsal part of the finger

Symbols, Signs, and Icons

For organizations such as the Boy Scouts of America and the University of Texas "Longhorns" to intricate physics concepts like the "left hand generator rule," fingers are used to form symbols that can represent countless entities and ideas, with all their connotations. These symbols do not always convey identical meanings across cultures (e.g. the extended middle finger), and may even overlap in connotation (e.g. raising two fingers can mean peace or victory and/or the number two). But overall, we rely heavily upon our fingers as a form of symbolic expression or as in icons, a statement of command, instruction, convenience, or contempt.

The source of the Vulcan salute

Though 1960s hippies misattributed the Vulcan salute first used in *Star Trek's* second season opening episode, "Amok Time," to a variation of the peace sign, the symbol is actually rooted in Jewish ritual. Leonard Nimoy, who plays the character Spock, drew upon the religious symbol used by the Kohanim, the descendents of Jewish priests. The now-ubiquitous gesture is still used in the "priestly blessing" performed on certain Jewish holidays – a ritual Nimoy was exposed to while attending synagogue as a child.

The hand figure is made by separating the hand into three parts: the thumb, index and middle finger, and then the ring finger and little finger. In Judaism, this symbol, representing the Hebrew letter "shin," standing for the name of G-d, is formed using both hands. The Vulcan salute, however, is expressed with one hand in the vertical position, making it more like a greeting.

In addition to their appearance, the two hand gestures also have similar meanings. Just as this sign is used during the priestly blessing by Kohanim, accepting G-d's blessing on behalf of the congregation, so too the Vulcan salute represents the phrase "live long and prosper." All in all, the Jewish implications of this otherwise secular salute are evident.

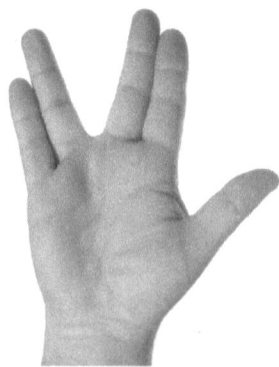

- **Crossing the fingers:**
  - crossing the middle finger over the index finger usually signifies a superstitious desire for good luck.

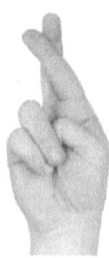

- **Raising 3 fingers:** Raising the index, middle, and ring finger on right hand

  - symbolizes the 3 parts of promise in the Boy and Girl Scouts of America

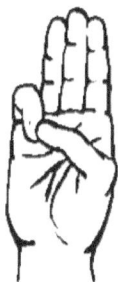

- **Raising the index and middle finger**

  - symbolizes peace
  - quiet
  - victory
  - number two
  - humorously in photographs to mean "bunny ears"
  - In the United Kingdom and New Zealand, making a "V" sign with the index and middle finger and the palm pointing towards you is the equivalent of the middle finger obscene gesture in the United States.

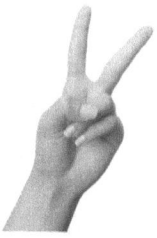

- **Sticking up the middle finger:**

  - obscene gesture and is also known as "flipping" or "flicking" someone off. The gesture of giving someone the middle finger is said to have originated in Ancient Greece where playwrights used the gesture as an insult in their writings, meant to symbolize the phallic disparagement used by primates. There has been a false historical reference about the middle finger relating to English archers and having their fingers cut off by the French during battle.

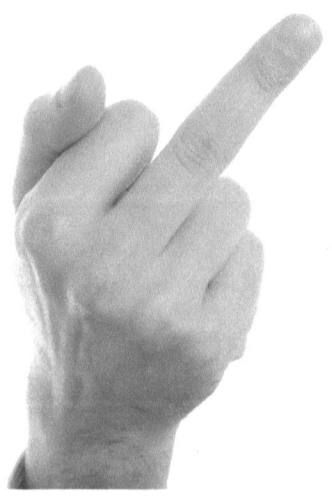

- **Thumbs up:**
  - Supportive gesture showing approval
  - In Iran, the thumb's up symbol is comparable to the middle finger obscene gesture in the United States.

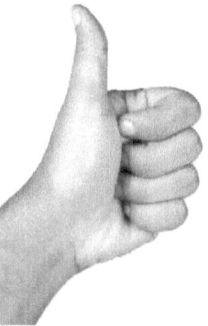

- **Thumbs down:**
  - Gesture showing disapproval

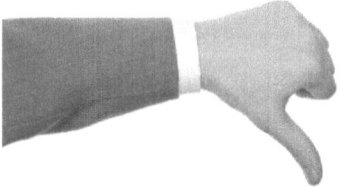

- **Index finger pointing upwards:**
  - showing direction

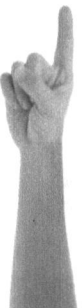

- **Left Hand Motor Rule in Physics:**
  - Used to determine the direction of the reaction force of a conductor with a current in a magnetic field. Place the thumb, index finger, and middle finger all perpendicular to each other. The index finger represents the direction of the

field, the thumb points in the direction of the movement of the conductor, and the middle finger points in the direction of the induced current.

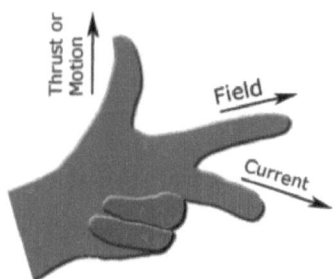

- **Right Hand Generator Rule in Physics:**
  - Used to determine the direction of the induced current of a conductor in a magnetic field. Place the thumb, index finger, and middle finger all perpendicular to each other. The index finger represents the direction of the field, the thumb points in the direction of the movement of the conductor, and the middle finger points in the direction of the induced current.

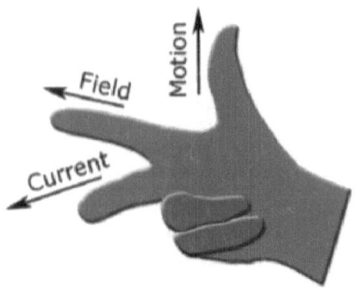

- **Jain Hand:**
  - symbol of the Jain religion
  - symbolizes nonviolence; the circle in the middle symbolizes a cycle and the word in the middle means "stop"; therefore, stopping the cycle of reincarnation and avoid hurting anything or anyone is the central theme.

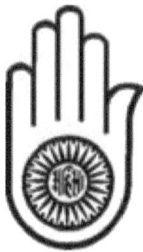

- **Healer's Hand:**
  - symbolizes energy healer hand of the Reiki

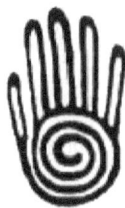

- **Hamsa:**
  - Symbol to protect against the evil eye

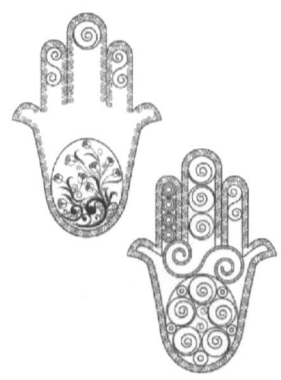

- **Raising the index and ring finger:**
  - Texas Longhorns
  - Rock star

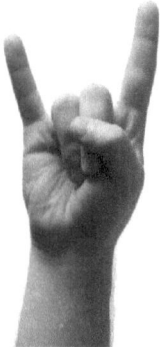

- **Making a "T" with both hands perpendicular:**
  - Timeout

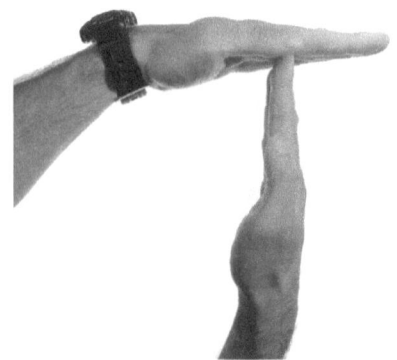

- **Tying a ribbon on the index finger:**
  - Reminder tactic

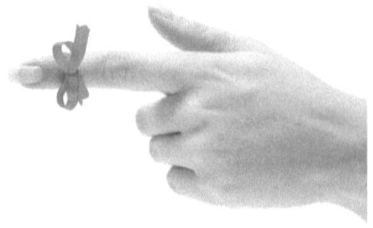

- **Placing palms of both hands together:**
  - Position used in prayer

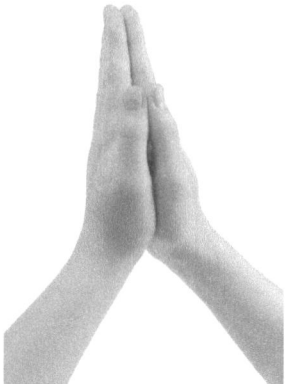

- **Interlocking little fingers with another person**
  - "pinky promise"

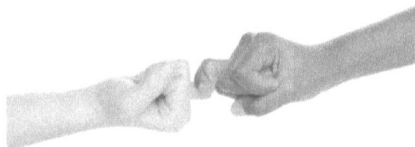

- **Raising middle, ring, and little fingers while thumb and index finger make a circle:**
  - "A-okay"; everything is going well

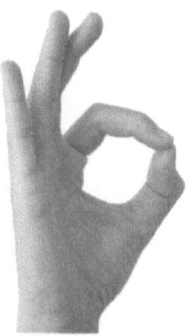

- **Open Hand**:
    - high five
    - saying hello

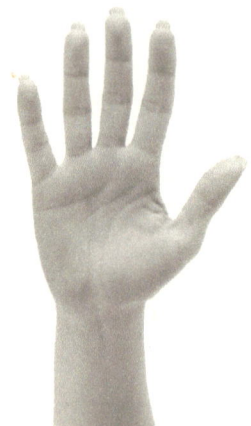

- **Index finger erect in one direction**:
    - pointing towards something or someone

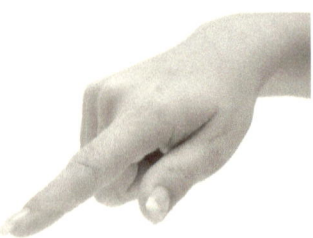

- **Index finger curled in toward hand**:
    - come here

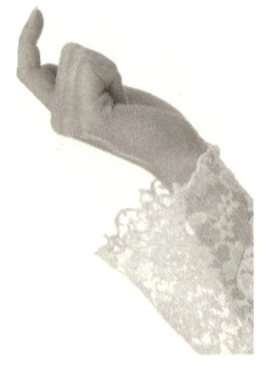

- **Index finger touching lips:**
  - Please keep quiet

TRIVIA

Cartoon Characters

Most cartoon characters on television and in movies are only drawn with three fingers and a thumb. Leaving a finger off of the drawings makes it much cheaper when the cartoon is being produced and it also makes it more aesthetically pleasing so the hand does not look so clustered. Some famous characters with only four digits are Mickey Mouse, Felix the Cat, and Bob the Builder.

In a quote by Homer Simpson on the show "The Simpson's," Homer comments on the birth of his son Bart Simpson and proclaims *"As long as he's got eight fingers and eight toes, he's fine by me!"*

Jewish Wedding Ritual

In Judaism, it is **customary for the groom to place the ring on the bride's index finger on the right hand,** as opposed to the ring finger on the left hand that is more traditionally used in Christianity. The explanation for this Jewish ritual is the ancient Talmudic belief that the index finger is closer to the heart because of a direct artery from that finger to the heart. The ring is usually moved to the ring finger after the ceremony.

Pinky Blessing

In Judaism, following the reading of the <u>Torah</u> in the Synagogue, it is customary to extend one's arm and pinky finger toward the Torah as it is lifted.

Snapping the fingers

In order to produce the sound known as "snapping," one must slide the middle finger rapidly passed the thumb and strike the palm of the hand.

Interesting articles highlighting the thumb:

Two articles in 2002 highlighted the growing concern that today's electronic gadgets are making the younger generation "all thumbs":

- An article in the *New York Post* on March 26, 2002 ("Phone, game studies a real thumb-dinger") cited the same research, saying of 21st century kids that today's gizmos "are changing the shape and dexterity of their fingers and thumbs" and have led to increased use of the thumb for tasks that were once performed by the other digits.

- According to an April 17, 2002 article in the *Wall Street Journal*, **thumbs have become the "universal index fingers for a generation of teenagers,** young adults and high-tech businesspeople" (A1). Thumbs are growing more muscled and dexterous, according to a cross-cultural study by free-lance British culture and technology researcher Sadie Plant. Additionally, our thumbs have traditionally enjoyed a wider range of motion than those of primates as well as our other digits, says Stanford University researcher Joseph Towles, who has studied thumb development for more than 25 years.

Press releases have cited similarly disturbing evidence of harm to the fingers and thumb caused by excessive use through text-messaging and similar methods of digital communication:

A 2002 Virgin Mobile press release found that 3.8 million people in the U.K. experience wrist and/or thumb pain as a result of text messaging.

The International Association for Wireless Communications said in a June 2007 press release that 158 billion text messages were sent in the year 2006 alone.

TYPING

There are numerous books available that teach people how to type. The Information Age mandates the use of typing skills in general and **QWERTY** keyboards in particular. Correct placement of the fingers is essential for efficient typing. **The classical instructions recommend that the little finger of the right hand should be on the semicolon key, the ring finger on the "L", the middle finger on the "K", the index finger on the "J", and the thumb on the space bar.** The left hand little finger should also be on the space bar. The left hand index finger on the "F", the middle finger on the "D", the ring finger on the "S", and the little finger on the "A".

WRONG SITE SURGERY

Wrong–site surgery is rare but shocking to the public.

Throughout the United States, reports suggest that surgeons may operate on the wrong site about 1,000 times a year.

In a survey of 1590 members of the American Society for Surgery of the Hand (ASSH), over 200 cases of wrong site surgery were reported: 128 of the fingers and 23 on the wrists.

Retrospectively, in 1969, in the second issue of a new British journal, Journal of Hand Surgery, Dr. H. Graham Stack, wrote a classic article, "Naming the Fingers", elaborating on these confusions, ambiguities, and misconceptions.

> The Secretary of the Medical Defence Union wrote in 1955: -
>
> .. "To do as many do--namely to number the fingers 1, 2, 3, etc. and to record in the clinical notes, for example, that finger number 3 requires amputation is to set the stage for a serious surgical mishap. Now and again the surgeon, reading the notes of the case at a later date, before proceeding to operate has counted wrongly by choosing to regard the thumb as number 1 instead of the index finger. In this way the wrong finger has been amputated or chosen for some other operation.

The Right Lessons From Wrong-Site Surgery

The error appears to have occurred because the team did not take a "time out" in the moment before the operation to ensure the "right patient, right procedure, right location."

> "It seems to the Council of the Union that this serious mistake would be obviated if hospital medical officers when writing up clinical notes described the actual finger affected by adopting the designations of "the thumb", "the index finger", "the middle finger", "the ring finger", and "the little finger".
>
> In September 1960 the Secretary of the Union again wrote reiterating this point in the same terms, as in the previous twelve months the Union had dealt with nine claims where an operation had been performed on the wrong limb or digit.
>
> In 1961 (and revised in 1966), a Joint Memorandum on Safeguards against wrong operations was produced by the Medical Defence Union, and the Royal College of Nursing, and the National Council of Nurses of the United Kingdom in which the following was written.
>
> ### Suggested safeguards
> **I.   In order to avoid the possibility of any ambiguity concerning the finger(s) on which the operation is to be performed, the fingers should always be described as thumb, index, middle, ring and little fingers, and not as 1st, 2nd, 3rd, 4th, and 5th.**

While various organizations and institutions, including the American Academy of Orthopaedic Surgeons, the American Association for Surgery of the Hand, and the Joint Commission (an independent organization that accredits and certifies health care organizations), have made various proposals and protocols to address this situation, the problem still exists and places a black mark on the medical profession.

Wrong site surgery mistakes are preventable if the proper standards of medical care are followed, and most cases are directly tied to human error and a failure to adhere to nationally recognized standards.

UNIVERSAL PROTOCOL

Accreditation Program: Ambulatory Health Care Chapter: National Patient Safety Goals[16]

1 For all procedures involving incision or percutaneous puncture or insertion, the intended procedure site is marked. The marking takes into consideration laterality, the surface (flexor, extensor), the level (spine), or specific digit or lesion to be treated.

> Note: For procedures that involve laterality of organs but the incision(s) or approaches may be from the mid-line or from a natural orifice, the site is still marked and the laterality noted.

2 The procedure site is initially marked before the patient is moved to the location where the procedure will be performed and takes place with the patient involved, awake and aware, if possible.

3 The procedure site is marked by a licensed independent practitioner or other provider who is privileged or permitted by the organization to perform the intended surgical or non-surgical invasive procedure. This individual will be involved directly in the procedure and will be present at the time the procedure is performed.

> Note: Final confirmation and verification of the site mark takes place during the time-out.

4 The method of marking the site and the type of mark is unambiguous and is used consistently throughout the organization.

5 The mark addresses the following:

- Is made at or near the procedure site or the incision site. Other non-procedure site(s) are not marked unless necessary for some other aspect of care.
- Includes, preferably, the surgeon's or proceduralist's initials, with or without a line representing the proposed incision.

---

16 Pre-Publication Version © The Joint Commission 2008

- Is made using a marker that is sufficiently permanent to remain visible after completion of the skin prep and sterile draping. Adhesive site markers are not to be used as the sole means of marking the site.

Hand Reflexology

Hand reflexology is the practice of placing pressure on the hands using certain finger and thumb massage techniques in order to heal other parts of the body. It is based on the belief that each part of the hand represents a different organ, muscle, or gland of the body.

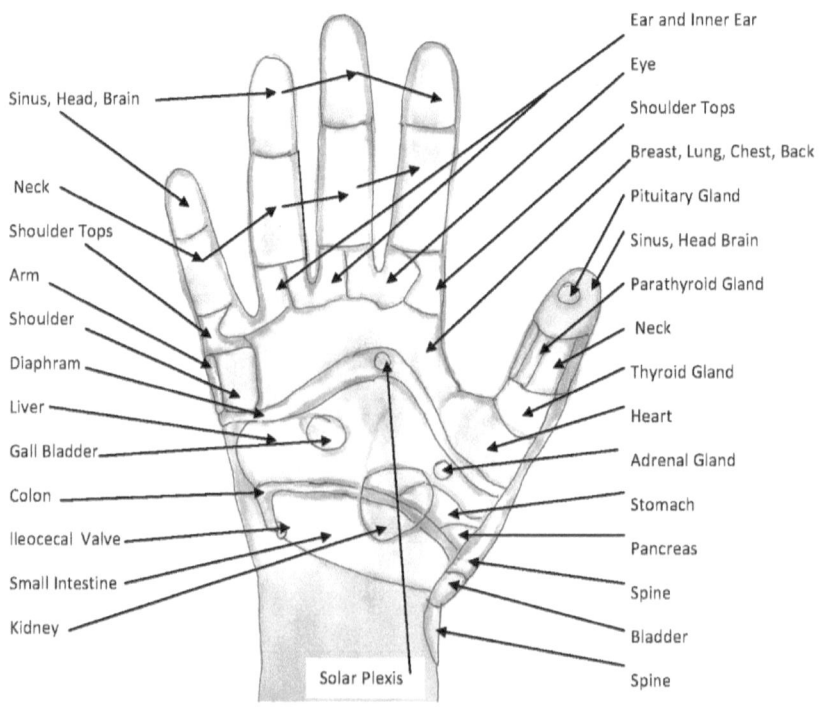

Ear and Inner Ear
Eye
Shoulder Tops
Breast, Lung, Chest, Back
Pituitary Gland
Sinus, Head Brain
Parathyroid Gland
Neck
Thyroid Gland
Heart
Adrenal Gland
Stomach
Pancreas
Spine
Bladder
Spine

Sinus, Head, Brain
Neck
Shoulder Tops
Arm
Shoulder
Diaphram
Liver
Gall Bladder
Colon
Ileocecal Valve
Small Intestine
Kidney

Solar Plexis

17

17 Courtesy of Lynne Pittard

About the Authors

Hillary J. Kener graduated Cum Laude with a Bachelor of Science from the University of Florida. She is currently pursuing a Master's Degree at The Johns Hopkins University. Her work has been featured in scientific journals and teen magazines alike. She enjoys fashion, fitness, and traveling, and has volunteered for numerous community service organizations over the years. She currently resides in Washington, D.C.

Michael Zeide, MD is an orthopedic surgeon in West Palm Beach, Florida. He is a past-president of the Florida Orthopedic Society and was an Clinical Associate Professor of Orthopedics for 20 years at the University of Miami. He is on the editorial board of the American Journal of Orthopedics. He is the co-author of the Orthopaedic Dictionary.

www.ingramcontent.com/pod-product-compliance
Lightning Source LLC
Chambersburg PA
CBHW032026170526
45157CB00002B/872